Type 1 Diabetes Caregiver Confidence

A Guide for Caregivers of Children Living with Type 1 Diabetes

Samantha Markovitz

Mayo Clinic Certified Wellness Coach

Author photography by Laura Pavlakovich of yourejustmytype.com.

Published by Prominence Publishing.
For information, visit www.prominencepublishing.com

Glucagon instructions reprinted with permission from Eli Lilly and Company.

Samantha Markovitz is the founder of GraceMark Wellness & Lifestyle Coaching. Samantha is also an in-demand speaker and consultant on issues relating to T1D.

Connect with Samantha Markovitz at www.T1Dcaregiverconfidence.com or www.gracemark.org.

ISBN: 978-0-9958274-2-4

What Others Are Saying...

As a teacher and potential type 1 diabetes caregiver, reading *Type 1 Diabetes Caregiver Confidence* provided the welcome reminder to always be prepared. I have gained vital knowledge regarding insulin delivery options, as well as the difference between sugar and carbohydrates as it pertains to T1D. As a result, I have created a classroom emergency kit, which includes an explanation of common symptoms of low blood sugar and a juice box.

I applaud Samantha in taking the step from supporting others by coaching individuals and families, to writing this book with the purpose of preventing in others the scares and life-threatening situations that T1D can present at its worst. Thank you for giving me the confidence that I need to approach my role as potential caregiver with strength and knowledge. *Type 1 Diabetes Caregiver Confidence* is a must-read for anyone working with children.

Linda Horist
2014 California Teacher of the Year

Ms. Markovitz provides a concisely written guide for those who will be caring for a child with diabetes. A type 1 diabetic herself, Samantha understands how complicated and confusing diabetes care can be. She has streamlined the information here, which will be a big help to those feeling overwhelmed by the prospect of caring for a child with type one diabetes.

Michelle Weisenberg
T1D Parent
Co-Founder, Project Blue November

The day our daughter was diagnosed at age 13 with T1D our world was turned upside down. What a blessing a book like this would have been to have for grandparents, teachers, school nurses, friends and even for us as parents! Thank you Samantha Markovitz for creating this essential tool for all who love and care for T1Ds!

Kristan Hinman
T1D Parent and Educator

Living with type 1 diabetes is tough. No one will ever tell you it's easy, but with the right knowledge, guidance and tools, it is a condition someone can live with very successfully. For those tasked with providing care for someone with type 1 diabetes (T1D), it can be an intimidating prospect. But, it doesn't need to be.

In *Type 1 Diabetes Caregiver Confidence*, Samantha Markovitz provides a comprehensive, easy to comprehend guide for understanding how to care for someone with T1D. When I first met Samantha shortly after her diagnosis with T1D, she was scared, uncertain and overwhelmed. In the years since then, she has educated herself, learned from her experiences and engaged with the T1D community, inspired to help those living with and affected by T1D in any way she can.

Type 1 Diabetes Caregiver Confidence is the embodiment of Samantha's desire to help the T1D community and will be a great tool to assist and empower those charged with caring for someone with T1D.

Michelle Popoff
Professional diabetes advocate
Diagnosed with T1D in October 1985

Acknowledgements

Thank you to the type 1 diabetes community for welcoming me with open arms upon my diagnosis in early young adulthood. I am forever grateful to belong to a club with the most wonderful people as members, even if the membership requirement is something we would all gladly return to sender, if it were possible. This book is for you, and the people who love and care for you.

Thank you to my family and friends for your love and support in my pursuit of this project.

A special thank you to those who shared their experience and broad perspectives while being my sounding board and wise counsel.

- ❖ Donna & Joel Markovitz
- ❖ Kristan & Sterling Hinman
- ❖ Sheila Glazov
- ❖ Rachel Schindelbeck
- ❖ Evan Markovitz
- ❖ Joan & Robert Lipson
- ❖ Kalee Hinman
- ❖ Michelle Popoff
- ❖ Anthony De Zan
- ❖ Juliet Gardner
- ❖ Faye Hanoian

About the Author

As a Mayo Clinic Certified Wellness Coach, Samantha Markovitz specializes in coaching and educating newly diagnosed families, while providing the support and materials needed to advocate for their child with type 1 diabetes.

As a person living with type 1 diabetes, she is uniquely qualified to provide support in dealing with the day-to-day challenges of life with T1D.

Vision and goal setting in relation to living well with diabetes is a large part of the coaching process. By considering the client to be the expert in their own life, Samantha assists in educating and advocating for them as individuals and families.

She is the founder of GraceMark Wellness & Lifestyle Coaching. Samantha is also an in-demand speaker and consultant on issues relating to T1D.

Foreword

Samantha Markovitz's *Type 1 Diabetes Caregiver Confidence: A Guide for Caregivers of Children Living with Type 1 Diabetes* is an exceptional book and resource that every parent and caregiver must have on their bookshelf. I definitely needed and would have treasured her book when our elder son was diagnosed with T1D in 1985.

Samantha's book offers parents and caregivers significant, relevant, and meaningful information about T1D. The book is precisely written in an easy to read format that is structured into 5 sections that you can reference as needed and not feel overwhelmed by too much new and/or unfamiliar T1D and medical information.

Samantha also includes "real life" experiences and information about the physical, emotional, and mental effects of T1D to help parents and caregivers maintain and encourage healthy diabetes management and reassuring well-being for children, parents, and caregivers.

Taking superb care of a child with T1D is challenging, but possible! As you read Samantha's book, you will discover how children with T1D can live healthy, joyful, normal lives, and achieve their heart's desire with balance and self-confidence. Yes, there will be good days and bad days that may be out of your control. However, you will learn to securely handle those unbalanced and unexpected situations, with the insightful education and skills this book provides.

After you read *Type 1 Diabetes Caregiver Confidence: A Guide for Caregivers of Children Living with Type 1 Diabetes*, you will know:

1. You are doing the best you can because you have the knowledge, tools, and abilities to help you understand the physical, psychological, and psychosocial effects of T1D.
2. You will be able to maintain good health, comfort, and self-assurance as a parent or caregiver.
3. You will become a confident T1D expert!

Sheila N. Glazov
Author of Purr-fect Pals: A Kid, A Cat and Diabetes
sheilaglazov.com/purr-fect-pal-diabetes-connection

Introduction

There are many books that have been written about diabetes. Out of all of those books about diabetes, very few focus on type 1 diabetes. Even fewer address a major cause of concern for parents of children with type 1 diabetes: how to feel confident leaving their child in the care of someone else.

Type 1 Diabetes Caregiver Confidence is the life-saving quick read you have been looking for since your child's diagnosis. We will cover all of the information your caregiver needs, without the intimidating details that are not relevant to their role. After reading this book, the caregiver(s) in your child's life will feel confident in their ability to care safely and compassionately for your child, and you will feel confident in knowing that your child is in good, well-informed hands in your absence.

This book is broken up into five sections.

Prior to Section 1, you will find the **Quick Reference** guide. Find the most important facts about caring for a child with type 1 diabetes (T1D) at your fingertips in these pages.

Section 1 - What is Diabetes?

- Covers fundamentals of your role as caregiver

- Provides a breakdown between type 1 and type 2 diabetes.

Section 2 - Diabetes Day-to-Day

- Examines the use of insulin and diabetes management tools (such as the glucometer, CGM, pump, MDI)

- Includes an overview of diabetes management tool function and practical use

- Covers strategies for handling situations such as snack time, physical activity, high blood sugar (hyperglycemia), low blood sugar (hypoglycemia), and the administration of Glucagon in an emergency

Section 3 - Caregiver Confidence

- Provides invaluable support and knowledge specific to caregivers with insight into special occasions

- Includes guidance in how to communicate effectively about T1D

- Discusses the complicated and varied emotions that can accompany T1D

- Encourages self-care and confidence in making a spirited effort to take on T1D

At the back of the book is the **Appendix**, which contains the fill-in **Caregiver Confidence Guide**, **Caregiver Conversation Guide**, followed by a **Glossary**. Caregivers can work with parents to fill in the vital information they need to have on hand, ranging from insulin dose ratios to emergency instructions.

At the beginning of each chapter, you will find a bulleted list. This is a brief summary of the chapter that includes important facts intended to help you access the information quickly, when you need it most.

Note: Throughout the book, you will see "T1D" used interchangeably with "type 1 diabetes" as shorthand to refer to type 1 diabetes as a disease, as well as to refer to a person who lives with type 1 diabetes.

Table of Contents:

T1D Caregiver Confidence
Quick Reference

Before we proceed to Section 1, I want to introduce you to the **T1D Caregiver Confidence Quick Reference**. Consider this the "flip-to-it" answer section that provides a quick reference for the absolute essentials needed in the moment, like recognizing the symptoms and treatment of low blood sugar. Detailed information on these topics can be found later on in the book, but in the moment, nothing beats having the facts at your fingertips, which is exactly what the **Quick Reference** pages are intended to provide.

Quick Reference Page	Topic	Where to find out more:
1	Commonly Asked Questions	*Type 1 Diabetes Caregiver Confidence*
2	#1 Thing to Look Out For: Low Blood Sugar	Chapter 8: Hypoglycemia/Low Blood Sugar
3	In Case of Extreme Low Blood Sugar: Use Glucagon	Chapter 9: In Case of Emergency: Administering Glucagon
4	High Blood Sugar + DKA	Chapter 10: Hyperglycemia/High Blood Sugar
5	Mobile Apps	App Store/Google Play

Type 1 Diabetes
Caregiver Confidence Quick Reference

Type 1 Diabetes Caregiver Confidence
Quick Reference

Commonly Asked Questions

Q: What does "T1D" mean?

A: T1D stands for "type 1 diabetes" and can be used as shorthand to refer to type 1 diabetes as a disease or someone who lives with type 1 diabetes.

Q: Is type 1 diabetes the same as juvenile or insulin dependent diabetes?

A: Yes; type 1 diabetes was formerly referred to as "juvenile " and "insulin dependent" diabetes. We now know that the onset of type 1 can occur at any age, and while ALL T1D individuals are dependent upon insulin, there are also some individuals with type 2 who require insulin as part of their diabetes management.

Q: What is the most important thing to know about keeping a child with T1D safe?

A: Low blood sugar (hypoglycemia) is the most immediate danger. Symptoms can include shakiness, sweating, weakness, irritability, dizziness, and hunger. Treatment is ingesting a source of fast-acting sugar.

Q: Is there anything a person with T1D cannot eat?

A: No; a person with T1D can eat anything as long as the carbohydrate content is accounted for with insulin, dosed per individual care plan. Consult with the parents to ensure the family is not subscribing to a special plan or dealing with an allergy or celiac disease in combination with T1D, which would require special attention.

Q: What do I need to do to take care of a child with T1D?

A: Consult with the parents of the child in your care to find out what the child's personal needs are, as every situation and individual is unique. The information in this book is intended to be helpful; it is not medical advice or clinical care, nor a substitute for either medical advice or clinical care. Diabetes mangement and experiences may vary greatly between individuals and families; the information covered in this book aims to touch upon a number of scenarios but is not an exhaustive or definitive guide.

See the **Confident Caregiver Guide** template in the **Appendix** for an information page for parents and/or medical team to fill out for the purpose of providing reference for caregiver(s).

Type 1 Diabetes Caregiver Confidence
<u>Quick Reference</u>

#1 Thing to Look Out For: Low Blood Sugar

If the T1D in your care is exhibiting symptoms of low blood sugar such as:

- Shakiness
- Dizziness
- Confusion
- Nausea
- Headache
- Slurred speech
- Impaired coordination

... they may be experiencing low blood sugar.

What happens next:

1. Know what blood glucose number the child's parents and/or medical team consider to be "low," then check blood sugar with a meter to confirm the symptoms with the resulting number

(General recommendation: 70 mg/dl or below – threshold may be higher or lower depending on the recommendation of the T1D medical team)

2. Treat low blood sugar IMMEDIATELY. Common treatment choices include a small juice box, glucose tablets, fruit snacks, or another quickly absorbed source of sugar

(General guideline: 15 grams fast-acting carbs every 15 minutes until blood sugar has returned to a safe level, as determined by the T1D medical team)

3. Follow up with a carb + protein snack to steady blood sugar

(Examples include peanut butter on toast, cheese and crackers, or graham crackers and milk)

More information available in Chapter 8: Hypoglycemia/Low Blood Sugar

Type 1 Diabetes Caregiver Confidence
Quick Reference

IN CASE OF EXTREME LOW BLOOD SUGAR
USE GLUCAGON

If your T1D is experiencing extreme low blood sugar and is unable or unwilling to receive sugar by mouth (example: unconscious, seizing, combative behavior, etc.), be prepared to use their prescribed Glucagon emergency kit.

Step 1: Flip off the seal from the vial of Glucagon powder.

Step 2: Remove the needle cover from the syringe. DO NOT REMOVE THE PLASTIC CLIP FROM THE SYRINGE, as this may allow the push rod to come out of the syringe.

Step 3: Insert the needle into the rubber stopper on the vial, then inject the entire contents of the syringe into the vial of Glucagon powder.

Step 4: Remove the syringe from the vial, then gently swirl the vial until liquid becomes clear. Glucagon should not be used unless the solution is clear and of a water-like consistency.

Step 5: Insert the same syringe into the vial and slowly withdraw all of the liquid. In children weighing less than 44 pounds, withdraw half of the liquid (0.5 mark on the syringe).

Step 6: Cleanse the buttock, arm, or thigh and inject Glucagon immediately after mixing, and then withdraw the needle. Apply light pressure against the injection site.

Step 7: Turn the person on his/her side. When an unconscious person awakens, he/she may vomit.

Call 911 immediately after administering Glucagon. If the person does not awaken within 15 minutes, you may administer a second dose of Glucagon, if previously instructed by your healthcare provider to do so.

Note: Glucagon may take 5-15 minutes to work

As soon as the person is awake and able to swallow, give him/her a fast-acting source of sugar (such as fruit juice), followed by a snack or meal containing both protein and carbohydrates (such as cheese and crackers, or a peanut butter sandwich).

Step 8: Discard any unused reconstituted Glucagon.

Remember to notify your healthcare provider that an episode of severe hypoglycemia has occurred.

These are not the complete instructions. Go to **Chapter 9: In Case of Emergency – Administering Glucagon** for complete instructions on how to administer Glucagon.

More information available in Chapter 9: In Case of Emergency – Administering Glucagon

Type 1 Diabetes Caregiver Confidence
<u>Quick Reference</u>

High Blood Sugar

If your T1D is exhibiting irritability, extreme thirst, tiredness, frequent need to use the restroom, or difficulty concentrating, they may be experiencing high blood sugar.

What happens next:

1. Check blood sugar with glucose meter to confirm

2. If result is over 250 mg/dl, test for ketones and do not allow exercise until below 250 mg/dl without ketones

3. Give corrective insulin dose according to individual care plan

4. Encourage non-caffeinated, sugar-free liquid intake (water recommended)

5. If high blood sugar persists, continue according to care plan provided by parents and/or medical team

Note: If the T1D is vomiting, having difficulty breathing, or showing confusion, call 911 immediately. He or she may be experiencing diabetic ketoacidosis, a life-threatening complication of T1D which requires immediate medical attention.

More information available in Chapter 10: Hyperglycemia/High Blood Sugar

Type 1 Diabetes Caregiver Confidence
Quick Reference

Mobile Apps

Glucagon by Eli Lilly and Company®

Essential information and instructions for administering a Glucagon injection in case of emergency low blood sugar, causing the T1D to be unable to swallow, unconscious, seizing, or uncooperative

MyFitnessPal®

Database of nutritional information and meal tracking capabilities

CalorieKing®

Database of nutritional information for grocery brands, fast food, and restaurant chains

Insulin Pumps and CGM

Each insulin pump and continuous glucose monitoring device manufacturer has their own app(s) with varied features which may include remote monitoring capabilities, FAQs, training videos, and access to customer care.

Section 1:
Diabetes Beginner Basics

CHAPTER 1:
THE ROLE OF A T1D CAREGIVER

- Taking on the role of type 1 diabetes (T1D) caregiver can be intimidating

- Feel empowered by your knowledge and level of preparedness

- Approach with strength

- Attempt a sense of normalcy

- Children sense your fear and frustration - try not to let them see you sweat

- Arm yourself with knowledge and extra supplies

- Learn from each day, in each moment, as it comes

- You've got this!

My philosophy of caregiving for type 1 diabetes, which I hope you will adopt or consider incorporating into your own, is about coming from a place of strength and hope, not fear and restriction. Caring for a child with diabetes can feel scary or intimidating. There is a lot of information out there, much of it outdated or simply inaccurate. Once you are armed with the correct information, in a concise format and digestible quantity, you will have the tools you need to help manage the diabetes of the T1D in your life.

Children with type 1 diabetes are just like other kids, except that they need guidance and support in the process of manually performing the tasks that replicate what was formerly handled by their pancreas. Unless the doctor or family has chosen a special diet that fits best for that child's unique needs, the menu for a T1D child should look like that of any other healthy, active child (including the occasional treat, which we all need every once in a while). He or she can participate in any sport or activity. It just requires a little more attention, particularly in regards to their blood glucose levels.

Your role as caregiver will vary a bit depending on the age of the child. For very young children, you will likely be responsible for every aspect of diabetes management (blood glucose level checking, food choices, carb counting, insulin dosing, monitoring for high/low blood sugar, etc.) while they are in your care. The age at which these tasks begin to transfer to the responsibility of the child may also vary. Having the T1D take the lead, while you mostly observe and jump in with hands-on help when needed, may be more appropriate for a mature pre-teen. For a teenager, cheering quietly from the sidelines might be the level of attention he/she needs from you. For a younger child or a teen that is experiencing burnout or other issues preventing him/her from focusing on the efficient and productive management of their diabetes, you may need to be more vocal and involved.

The most helpful advice I can give you is to be prepared. My mom always told me to carry an umbrella, even on the slightest chance that it might rain, because it was better to have it and not need it, than to need it and not have it. My point here is that it is better to be equipped with information and supplies and not ever need to use it than to realize, at the worst possible time, you need to know more or have more in that pivotal moment.

It never hurts to have back up supplies or a back up plan. This can mean different things to different people. It could be as simple as a teacher keeping an extra juice box in his/her desk, a school nurse keeping an extra meter kit in the office (store brands easily accessible at big box stores), a playmate's parent knowing the signs of a pump failure, or grandparents keeping a dedicated Glucagon kit at their house for sleepovers.

You are going to have many questions. The answer to many of your questions will be "it depends." The reality that there are few concrete answers will frustrate you. There is not an exact formula for your desired results. They say managing diabetes is not just a science, but a fine art, as well. Every child and adult with type 1 diabetes is a unique individual, and his/her diabetes may vary. This means a solution from a friend or the internet may not work for your child, or even a strategy that has been successful for his/her own diabetes management in the past may not work today or tomorrow (but maybe next month it will again—you never know!). The important thing is to keep perspective and maintain hope, especially when T1D is giving you trouble.

When we come from, and live in, a place of strength and hope, we create possibilities and embrace a future full of light and wonder. When we come from, and live in, a place of fear and restriction, we are closed off, sad, and have trouble even imagining a future, let alone one where wonderful things can and will happen. Choosing that place of strength and hope is not always easy, but it is worthwhile and achievable.

As a caregiver, it will be important that you remember to come from that place of strength and hope, especially when there are tough days (because there will be tough days). Not only will you need it for your own well-being and self-care, but also because you will be caring for someone who is looking to you and the other adults in their life to encourage stability and confidence while managing their diabetes.

You can do this. If you are not already doing it, you will begin today.

CHAPTER 2:
WHAT IS DIABETES?

Type 1 diabetes	Type 2 diabetes
• Autoimmune disease	• Metabolic condition
• No method of prevention	• Strong genetic component
• No cure	• Often develops later in life
• May be diagnosed at any age, though often diagnosed in childhood	• May develop due to lifestyle risk factors
• Treatment <u>always</u> includes insulin therapy	• The pancreas still creates insulin, but struggles to utilize it properly or produce the amount needed, due to insulin resistance
• People with this chronic condition <u>must</u> inject or pump insulin into the body to survive, as the pancreas no longer creates insulin	• Treatment may begin with diet and exercise, then progress to oral medications, non-insulin injectables, and/or insulin

You are reading this book because someone close to you lives with type 1 diabetes (T1D), or you have been asked to care for a child with T1D. Caregivers, I am going to help you learn what you need to know in a way that prevents unease and builds your type 1 diabetes caregiver skills. Let's start by answering the very common questions that people have when presented with the proposition of watching over a child who lives with diabetes.

"What is diabetes?"

"What is the difference between type 1 and type 2 diabetes?"

If you watch television, read magazines, or go on the internet, it is likely that you have heard or seen the word "diabetes" in an advertisement or article that was referring to type 2 diabetes.

Type 2 diabetes is a metabolic condition that occurs when the body becomes insulin resistant and the pancreas can no longer keep up production of the necessary amount of insulin. In this situation, the body either is not creating enough insulin to keep up with increased insulin needs due to insulin resistance, or it is unable to utilize the naturally produced insulin properly in order to maintain normal blood glucose levels.

The disease that we are focusing on in this book is **type 1 diabetes**.

Type 1 diabetes is an autoimmune disease that attacks the pancreas' production of insulin, a hormone essential to the body's ability to use glucose for energy. There is no way to prevent developing type 1 diabetes and thus far, there is no cure. Our task is to manage blood glucose levels using the technology that research has created while we await a biological cure. We strive to build an atmosphere where life for the person with type 1 diabetes is interrupted by the disease as infrequently as possible, while managing their blood glucose with the goal of safely keeping levels as close to target as possible.

In the United States of America, type 1 diabetes is a federally protected disability, as it meets the criteria of disruption to a major life function. The Americans with Disabilities Act (sometimes referred to as the ADA, not to be confused with the American Diabetes Association, which is also known as the ADA) protects people with type 1 diabetes, as the interruption to the essential functions of the endocrine system takes away the ability to function without medical intervention.

Many families make a conscious choice to not think of type 1 diabetes as a disability, if they find that it helps them to feel more empowered. Individuals with type 1 diabetes are capable of living an otherwise healthy existence, full of life's joys. While the distinction of T1D as a disability is what allows children with type 1 diabetes access to the modifications/accommodations needed to be safe and healthy out in the world, at daycare, school, camp, and one day, in their workplace, it does not mean that people with T1D are any less capable.

Section 2:
Diabetes Day-to-Day

CHAPTER 3:
WHAT CAUSES BLOOD GLUCOSE FLUCTUATIONS?

- There are many causes of blood glucose fluctuations

- Almost any internal or external factor can influence blood glucose management

- Stay calm and anticipate these changes whenever possible

- Use your knowledge and the tools at hand to ride the blood sugar rollercoaster

- Even out peaks and valleys in glucose levels whenever possible

When I was first diagnosed with type 1 diabetes, I had a difficult time finding a healthcare team that truly understood type 1 diabetes and could provide the knowledge and support that a newly diagnosed T1D requires (for example, the kind of information I hope you might be gleaning from this book). On my quest, I had an appointment with a Certified Diabetes Educator (CDE) from my local healthcare system.

She looked at me with a polite smile and said, with a note of impatience, "This is easy. All you need to know is that when you eat carbs, your blood sugar will go up, and when you take insulin, your blood sugar will go down. That's it."

What we would give to have it be that easy, right? What I didn't know then, that I know now, which you will now know as well, is that the answer to the question, "What causes blood glucose fluctuations?" is a two-word answer that is anything but simple.

That two-word answer is: "It depends."

Here are just a few examples of what might cause blood sugar to swing in one direction or the other (by no means an exhaustive list):

Cause of Low Blood Sugar	Cause of High Blood Sugar
Overestimating mealtime insulin dose	Underestimating mealtime insulin dose
Basal rate or long-acting insulin dose too high	Basal rate or long-acting insulin dose too low
Physical activity – cardio	Physical activity – strength training
Physical activity - chores	Puberty
Skipping a meal or snack after taking insulin to eat	Menstrual cycle

Cause of Low Blood Sugar	Cause of High Blood Sugar
Eating less carbs than appropriate for amount of insulin taken	Insulin degradation/improper storage/expiration
Stacking insulin doses	Pump site failure/pump occlusion (air bubble in tubing)
Delayed absorption of carbohydrates	Dehydration
Vomiting (inability to absorb carbs consumed)	Extended periods of being sedentary (lengthy car rides, academic testing, etc.)

"It Depends"
May raise or lower blood sugar depending on the individual or circumstance
Physical stress/illness
Emotional stress
Hot/cold weather
Hormonal fluctuation
Altitude changes
Lack of sleep
Exposure to direct sunlight
Prescription or OTC medications
Rate of absorption at site of insulin injection or infusion

Correcting Blood Sugar Fluctuations – The Basics

If blood sugar is fluctuating downward, the quickest solution is to eat a snack. If it is trending towards, or already rapidly approaching, low blood sugar, treat with a fast-acting source of sugar (see **Chapter 8 – Low Blood Sugar/Hypoglycemia**).

If blood sugar has fluctuated upward, it may be time to deliver a correction dose of insulin to bring the number back into the desired range. The amount of rapid-acting insulin needed to bring blood glucose back down into the target range is called a correction factor. It may be expressed in a ratio. Refer to the directions from the parents and/or medical team to find the correction factor that is tailored to the child in your care as well as in which situations to administer.

Remember – The insulin analogs that are available to people with type 1 diabetes are not as fast acting as naturally produced insulin, which means that the timing of the food and insulin may not always match up. This means you may see post-meal (post-prandial) spikes that will tempt you to correct, but it is often wise to wait and see how the insulin on board (IOB) works once it kicks in. This can also mean that you may see a dip in blood glucose after eating if the insulin becomes active before the food is metabolized. Ask the parents and/or medical team how they recommend dealing with these post-meal situations.

Example: With a correction factor of 1:60, it takes one unit of insulin to lower my blood sugar by 60 points. I will need to calculate how many points above my target number (let's use 120) and divide by 60 to discover how many units I need to take to reach 120. By this calculation, in order to correct a high blood glucose result of 240, I will need to take two units of rapid-acting insulin to reach my target number of 120.

1 unit of insulin to lower blood sugar by 60 points (correction factor 1:60)

With a current BG of 240 and a target of 120, I will subtract the target from current:

240-120=120

Then I will divide the result, 120, by my correction factor of 60

120/60=2

The result is the number of units (2) I will deliver to correct my blood sugar from 240 to 120

Note: Blood glucose fluctuations that result from illness and/or vomiting are very serious and require close monitoring. Not being able to keep food down after taking insulin can result in dangerously low blood sugar. A physical stress reaction to fighting illness can cause high blood sugar. Blood ketones can become a concern. Hydration is vital in either case.

Even something that may seem minor, like a common cold or flu, has the potential to put a child with type 1 diabetes in the hospital. Please be mindful about spreading germs by keeping clean surfaces, washing hands, receiving a flu shot, and implementing other standard illness prevention measures. Your efforts are much appreciated. Remember to go over your sick day plan with the child's parents and/or medical team so you will be prepared in case the child falls ill while under your care.

CHAPTER 4:
HOW TO USE A GLUCOSE METER

- A glucose meter may also be called a glucometer; also commonly referred to as simply a "meter"

- A meter is a portable medical device that must always be with the T1D, along with compatible test strips and lancing device

- It evaluates the level of glucose present in a drop of blood placed on a test strip inserted into the device

- This is a vital and necessary tool because insulin dosing decisions and fast-acting carb treatments for lows are dependent upon knowing the blood sugar number that the meter presents

- Tip: If you are ever in a situation where you and the child are out and about and have misplaced or forgotten the meter, Wal-Mart and Target both make inexpensive meters and less expensive strips that are available over the counter to help in a pinch

Tools necessary for glucose meter use include:

- glucose meter

- compatible test strips

- lancing device with loaded lancet

- alcohol swab/hand cleansing wipe

Each meter uses test strips that are designed specifically for that model of meter. Meter strips are not interchangeable. Use the companion strips for the meter, which are to be discarded after one-time use.

Begin by inserting a strip into the slot on the device. The test strips have receptor spots on the sides and/or end of the strip. Using a lancet in a spring-loaded lancing device, a small blood sample will be drawn. This process, resulting in a small gauge pin poking the fingertip to draw a tiny amount of blood, may be referred to as a fingerstick. The blood sample will be held up to one of the strip receptor spots until the meter acknowledges that it is reading the sample. Do not remove the strip from the meter until analysis is complete. When the meter is done analyzing the blood sample, it then produces a number result, which you will use to make blood glucose management decisions, based on the child's diabetes management plan.

In the US, blood glucose levels are measured in milligrams per deciliter (mg/dL). In Europe and Canada, blood glucose levels are measured in millimoles/liter (mmoL/L). We will talk about blood glucose levels in mg/dL, but if you reside in a country where mmoL/L is the standard of measurement, there are websites and mobile apps that provide a quick converter calculator that you can refer to if needed.

Note: 1 mmoL = 18 mg/dL

Each glucose meter will vary a bit in how to operate, so be sure to refer to the manufacturer instruction guide if you are not familiar. However, most meters are fairly intuitive to use, so do not be too concerned about messing something up.

Note: Meters run on either batteries or a charge, so be mindful of keeping back up power sources on hand.

A quick note about the fingerstick blood draw process. Everyone wants to know--does it hurt? Sometimes, but usually it is not very painful, thanks to the small gauge lancets that are now available. Painful or not, this is a crucial piece of diabetes management, so it must be done. Children may go through phases where they find this act more traumatic, either because their little fingers are more sensitive or they feel frustrated, intimidated, or simply perceive it as painful or unfair. At other times, the child may impress you with their nonchalant attitude towards just getting it done so they can get back to whatever it was they were doing beforehand.

Children with T1D test their blood sugar multiple times a day. This is routine for them; it is necessary for their health. It is critical to show sincere empathy and to encourage them not to be scared or upset. Acknowledge their feelings and emotions.

Think about when a child is learning to walk and they stumble. They usually wait to see what the adult response is ("Oh no! Are you okay?" vs. "Oops! Let's get back up and try again!") before they react and apply the emotions as a filter on future experiences. High-five them, make jokes, applaud their good attitude; try not to make a point of reminding them of how their peers do not have to go through the same process, how painful others may perceive the process to be, or say things like "Gosh, I don't know how you do that 10 times a day! I couldn't do it."

The reality is that you could, and would, do it if it meant keeping yourself alive. This is how and why children, and their parents and caregivers, continue to check blood sugar multiple times a day, even when it is somewhat unpleasant and uncomfortable.

Occasions that require a glucose check:

- Upon waking
- Before eating
- Before giving insulin
- Before treating low blood sugar
- Before physical activity
- During physical activity
- After physical activity
- Before sleep
- Before driving
- When alarms on CGM or remote monitoring apps indicate that there is a low or high
- If the child feels unwell or exhibits unusual behavior
- Any time that anything seems "off" to you, as the caregiver

The Step-by-Step Quick Guide to Using a Glucose Meter

1. Before checking the child's blood sugar level, make sure that both you and the child have clean hands. Residue from snacks, lotions, or other substances can skew the readings, so it is important to wash with soap and water, or use hand wipes, if possible. Alcohol swabs are also an option for cleaning the test site. If you will be handling the test strips, it is important that your hands are also clean, for the same reason.

2. Load the lancet in the lancing device and adjust for appropriate depth of lancing, which will vary by individual.

3. Insert a compatible test strip into the strip port on the meter. When the meter screen indicates that it is ready, prepare the blood sample.

4. Place the lancing device on the side of a finger pad and release the lancing function. If a droplet of blood is not present, squeeze the finger gently until one appears.

5. Line the blood drop up with the target spot on the test strip. Depending on the strip style, the target spot(s) will either be on the end or sides of the strip.

6. The meter will indicate that it is processing the blood sample. **Do not remove the strip while it is still processing** (removing the strip may disrupt the process and force you to start over with a new strip). Many people do not realize that the quantities of these essential one-time use strips are limited by insurance. They may be tiny, but they can be quite expensive, so do your best to avoid unnecessary waste.

7. When the meter is done processing the blood sample, it will show a number on the screen. That number represents the amount of glucose present in the blood at that moment in time.

8. If the child uses a digital or paper logbook, this would be the time to record the number result, as well as notes about carb intake, activities, or other details.

9. Using the target and treatment guidelines set by your T1D's parents and doctors, evaluate the next step and take action as appropriate.

If the number is **lower** than the target, a snack and/or fast-acting sugar should be given.

If the number is **higher** than the target, deliver a correction dose of insulin based on the correction factor as directed by the parents and/or medical team. Take into account any recent or upcoming physical activity, which may also lower glucose levels.

If the number is **within** the target range, celebrate! Even with the most careful and diligent management strategy, it is a rare snapshot in time, so enjoy the moment.

Keep in mind that correcting blood glucose too soon after eating does not give the active insulin on board the opportunity to peak and see its job through from dose to digestion. This is called "stacking" insulin, and can be very dangerous. Be sure to get a clear explanation from your T1D's parents and/or medical team regarding what the circumstances and directions are for his/her corrective insulin doses.

Target numbers and ranges vary by individual, especially when taking age into consideration. The younger a child is, the higher their target range is likely to be since the main goal would be to avoid dangerous episodes of low blood sugar, which can be more difficult to detect when a child is too young to express what they are feeling. As always, consult with the parents and/or medical team in order to know what the safe goals are for your T1D.

Remember that, despite the best efforts of all involved, sometimes blood glucose readings result in numbers that are outside of target range. Choose to regard this data as just that: information. That is why we try to remember to call it "checking" blood sugar instead of "testing." There is no right or wrong number, just in-range and out-of-range; information that helps us make our next diabetes management decision. If necessary, we correct. Then we move on.

CHAPTER 5:
HOW TO USE A CONTINUOUS GLUCOSE MONITOR (CGM)

- Continuous glucose monitoring systems (CGM) provide a continuous stream of glucose readings, every five minutes

- Data comes from a sensor wire inserted under the skin, transmitted to either a receiver and/or cellular phone application

- The HIGH/LOW threshold alarms help keep the user safe by alerting to out-of-range values

- Trend data and arrows help to provide a full picture of diabetes management

- The data viewer is empowered by CGM to make decisions regarding treatment in context, not just one moment in time (versus data from a fingerstick glucose meter check alone)

- Remember: you must still verify CGM BG data with a fingerstick meter check

Now considered an element of the standard of modern diabetes care, a continuous glucose monitor (CGM) is a valuable addition to traditional fingerstick glucose testing. While a glucose meter captures glucose level data from one moment in time, a continuous glucose monitor offers a new data point every five minutes to keep you informed between fingerstick checks. Directional trend arrows provide context for the direction in which the blood glucose levels are heading, accompanying the frequent data delivered every five minutes. Programmable high and low alert settings assist in notifying you when glucose levels are out of range. The period of time that is FDA-approved for CGM sensors is called a "sensor session."

There are patients who do not wear or utilize CGM for a variety of reasons, so this section only applies if your T1D has made CGM a part of their diabetes management plan.

Although CGM is fairly accurate, they do often have a lag time, especially when encountering major blood sugar swings. They may also be less accurate if not calibrated regularly in accordance with manufacturer directions. It is considered best practice to check a CGM number against a meter reading before making a treatment decision.

At the time of this publication, there are currently two manufacturers of CGM systems in the US: Dexcom® and Medtronic®. Systems made by both Dexcom and Medtronic can stand alone and work independently for use with either MDI (multiple daily injections) or insulin pump therapy. There are also some pumps that are integrated with CGM, such as the Animas® Vibe (Dexcom), Tandem® T-Slim (Dexcom), and MiniMed® 530G/630G/670G (Medtronic). Dexcom and Medtronic CGM each have unique features, but they both collect data from sensors that have small wires inserted and worn under the skin for days at a time. CGM systems require calibration data from fingerstick glucose testing (via glucose meter).

The elements of a continuous glucose monitoring system are:

- Sensor

- Transmitter (good for 3-12 months depending on the model—**do not dispose**)

- Receiver (in some systems, receiver hardware may be duplicated or replaced by a mobile app on a phone and/or smart watch)

Depending on what model of CGM system your T1D is using, you may have the ability to monitor their glucose levels from a distance on your phone or a smart watch, using apps like Dexcom Share or a variety of user-informed options from Nightscout.

Examples of how to utilize data from CGM in making treatment and management decisions:

Ex. 1: Low

CGM shows reading of 80, with a trending down arrow. Check with meter to verify. If the number is accurate, you will likely want to give a snack or (depending on how quickly the number is dropping and the medical care plan set in place for the T1D) begin treating with a source of fast-acting carbohydrates, backed up by a protein/fiber snack.

Ex. 2: High

CGM shows reading of 250, with a trending up arrow. Check with meter to verify. If the number is accurate, test for ketones (see **Chapter 11 – Hyperglycemia**), and evaluate if a correction bolus is appropriate at this time. Take into consideration IOB (insulin on board [active insulin] from the most recent previous bolus).

Ex. 3: Physical Activity

Keeping the CGM receiver or mobile data on-hand for quick reference during exercise or heightened physical activity will help you and your T1D stay aware of the direction blood glucose levels are going. If numbers begin to decline, you can provide a sip of sports drink or juice before it becomes an emergency. If the line is steady, you get peace of mind knowing that the child can safely proceed with their activity. If the numbers begin to creep up, you can keep an eye on that and see if it will need further action later. Since blood sugar drops related to physical activity can happen many hours later, CGM will help monitor stability and safety in these times as well.

Note: Some people experience post-exercise highs, especially after strength and conditioning. Sometimes waiting to see if the numbers begin to correct themselves is the safer option, as overcorrecting may cause dangerous lows later. Consult with the parents and/or medical team regarding desired treatment in this situation.

Ex. 4: Inaccurate data

If the CGM alerts for a number that you or the T1D do not feel is accurate, proceed by verifying with a meter. If the number on the glucose meter is different from the one on the CGM screen, go with the number from the meter fingerstick. Depending on the CGM directions, you may enter the blood glucose value to calibrate the system. If the CGM provides vastly inaccurate readings for a period of time, inform the parents so that they may call the manufacturer to report the failure and replace the sensor with a new one. Keep in mind that regular calibration is essential to keeping the CGM reading accurately. You may experience lag time between large blood sugar swings.

Troubleshooting for CGM

If you find that the sensor is coming off of the T1D before the sensor session is complete, clean the surrounding area with an alcohol swab. Carefully trim any of the sensor adhesive that has peeled up, then cover with your choice of medical tape products that will protect and keep the CGM sensor site in place until the conclusion of the sensor session. Avoid taping over the transmitter, covering just the adhesive edges of the sensor.

Reason(s) for Inaccurate Data or Error	Troubleshooting Recommendation
Dehydration	Drink water
Out of communication range	Place transmitter and receiver within 20 feet of each other and remove any obstructions (walls, etc.) Bathing or swimming may affect communication range as well.
Sensor compression	Reposition user to remove pressure on the sensor (ex: child laying on sensor site while sleeping)
Medications containing acetaminophen	Rely solely on fingerstick blood glucose meter tests until the acetaminophen runs its course
Improper storage of sensors	Report sensor to manufacturer and replace with a sensor that was stored between 36-77 degrees Fahrenheit
Significant glucose rise/fall in a short period of time	Rely on fingerstick results until the major swing has subsided; be sure to calibrate during periods of stable glucose levels

If the CGM is malfunctioning and needs to be replaced, inform your T1D's parents promptly. They may call the manufacturer or, depending on your role, ask you to call the manufacturer to report the device failure and to receive further instruction on how to get a replacement for the malfunctioning component as quickly as possible.

CHAPTER 6:
HOW TO WORK WITH INSULIN

- Insulin is a hormone

- Produced by the pancreas, or in the case of people with type 1 diabetes, it is injected or pumped into the body

- Enables the body to utilize glucose for energy

- Without insulin, the body loses the ability to utilize glucose for energy, eventually wasting away

- Ways to receive insulin therapy are injection by syringe, insulin pen, or insulin pump, of which there are various models on the market

Insulin is a hormone that is produced naturally by the body in the pancreas, under normal circumstances. Since people with type 1 diabetes are no longer capable of producing insulin, it is up to the individual and/or their caregiver to facilitate the measurement and administration of insulin to make up for the disrupted endocrine process.

At this point, we know what function insulin serves in the body ("unlocking" the ability for glucose to be absorbed into the cells for energy). We also know that people with type 1 diabetes no longer have the ability to produce their own insulin. This means that T1Ds need to mimic this process, by either injecting or pumping insulin into the body, subcutaneously (under skin, into fat). There may be no choice about needing to get insulin in the body, but there is a choice on how to get that insulin in there. There are two ways to do this: multiple daily injections (MDI) or insulin pump therapy. Both strategies, when utilized to the fullest potential, can provide a means to well-managed diabetes.

There are numbers and medical outcomes associated with what might be considered "well-managed" diabetes in a clinical sense. In this case, consider well-managed diabetes to look like a happy, healthy kid living a life with minimal interruptions due to chronic disease. T1D is an incredibly personal disease, so everyone has to give their insulin delivery plan serious thought and consideration in order to choose what works best for them in the context of their own life.

Multiple Daily Injections (MDI)

With MDI, there are two types of insulin that are injected. Rapid-acting insulin (such as Humalog®, NovoLog®, or Apidra®) is given by pen or syringe for meals, snacks, and corrections. Long-acting insulin (such as Lantus® or Levemir®) is injected once (or twice for a split dose) daily as an essential complement to fast-acting insulin.

Giving fast-acting insulin is called a bolus (or "bolusing"), while long-acting insulin is referred to as basal insulin. Both types of insulin are essential for a T1D on MDI. No exceptions.

Multiple Daily Injections (MDI) Supplies:

1. Alcohol swabs for preparing injection site

2. Fast-acting insulin (either vials or pens—yes, plural... always have a back up!)

3. Long-acting insulin (vials or pens, even if you think you'll be home in time for the long-acting dose; we never know when plans can change)

Note: Insulin needs to be kept out of extreme temperatures; if you anticipate extreme heat, take steps to keep the vial or pen cool. Extreme heat or cold can cause the insulin to lose potency.

4. Syringes (keep more than you think you need with you)

5. Pen needle caps (again, keep more than you think you need—allow for the occasional broken or bent needle in the bunch)

6. Method of needle disposal (sharps container or secure storage to accumulate sharps until a sharps container is available—small Tupperware or a plastic gum box also work well)

Syringes and pen needle caps should only be used once and then disposed of in a sharps container. If you are unable to locate a sharps container, a sandwich "trash" bag or small container to collect diabetes trash until you are near a sharps container will do just fine. Some families also use designated empty laundry detergent bottles or drink bottles to safely store used sharps. Disposing of sharps properly is important for preventing needlestick injuries from handling needles after use.

There are handy tools that can help with things like remembering doses and tracking the most recent dose when using MDI:

Timesulin® insulin pen replacement caps:

- Available online and at select retail locations, these caps begin tracking time elapsed between pen use the second you replace the cap on the pen.

- It is easy to forget whether you have given insulin or not, so the assistance of these caps can be invaluable, enabling you to refer back to see how long it has been since the last dose.

- There are now insulin pens in development that may have this type of tracking feature built-in, so you may see these smart features, including some that connect to a mobile app, utilized by insulin manufacturers going forward.

Mobile phone apps:

- Let your smartphone take some of the smaller tasks of diabetes care off of your shoulders.

- For example, many glucose meters now have Bluetooth® technology and a corresponding phone app that helps function as a bolus calculator. This is a great tool for MDI users, since it provides many of the features that pump therapy offers, including insulin on board (IOB) calculations, basal dose alarms and recording, and help on activity-based dosing adjustments, like exercise or recent hypoglycemia/low blood sugar.

- Keep in mind that if you choose to use an app that is not associated with an FDA-approved device, it may not be regulated for accuracy.

Insulin Pump Therapy

With insulin pump therapy, fast-acting insulin is used for both bolus and basal dosing. The one exception to this is "untethered" pumping, which is when the T1D receives their basal insulin from a long-acting insulin injection and uses the pump to bolus for food or corrections only.

The user programs their dosing formulas into the pump, which utilizes the pre-programmed ratios and insulin on board (IOB) calculators to present the user with a suggested dose for the proper amount of insulin for meals, snacks, or corrections. Unlike MDI, the basal insulin is not delivered through long-acting insulin like Lantus or Levemir. The basal insulin dose (also known as "basal rate") instead comes from the fast-acting insulin already in the pump, delivered in micro-doses 24 hours a day.

There are a few different pump manufacturers and models available at this point in time; each product has varied features and user interface, but the main function of facilitating the delivery of insulin is present in every one.

Ask for a written copy of formulas needed to calculate insulin dosage, including insulin to carb ratio, correction factor, basal rate/basal dose and insulin action time. It will be important to keep this information on hand in case of a pump malfunction that could erase stored data. It is helpful if you can take note of unusual reactions or what may seem to constitute a pattern, in regards to insulin dosage. Provide notes of unusual reactions or emerging patterns to the parents so they or their medical team can tweak insulin dosage.

CHAPTER 7:
FOOD: MACRONUTRIENTS AND MAKING CHOICES

- Children living with T1D can eat anything any other child can eat (barring any unique food directives or special dietary needs as stated by the parents and/or medical team)

- Carbohydrates are accounted for with insulin ("carb counting") dosed per the child's insulin to carb ratio

- Fat, protein, and carbohydrates are the macronutrients that make up our diets and can be used to plan balanced meals

- Sugar-free does not mean carb-free

- Sugar-free foods are not good substitutes as they can cause gastrointestinal distress

- If celiac disease or gluten sensitivity is in play, be sure to watch for sneaky sources of gluten when planning meals/snacks, or while eating out

- Remember that in the case of low blood sugar, fast-acting sugars such as juice, regular soda, or candy are a life-saving treatment

- **Never deny sugar in a low blood sugar emergency**

This chapter is about the diabetic diet.

Just kidding! There is no such thing as "the diabetic diet." Before the flexibility and knowledge afforded to us today by progressive research and insulin analogs, there were far more restrictions on what someone with diabetes would need to eat or avoid eating in order to manage their diabetes well. Today, we no longer deal with the regimented diets, exchange systems, or precisely timed meals and snacks that were the norm even just 20 years ago, before fast-acting insulin came on the scene for patient use.

Right away, we need to dispel the myth that people who live with type 1 diabetes cannot eat sugar. Not only is that not true, but during cases of hypoglycemia or low blood glucose (sugar), a fast-acting source of glucose (often delivered in the form of juice, regular soda, or candy) is a quick and necessary lifesaver.

You know that fast-acting carbs can mitigate or prevent a scary situation. Here are some examples of items to keep on hand or look for in case of emergency:

Treatment	**Serving**	**Carb Count**
Juicy Juice® Fruit Punch	4.23 oz	15 carbohydrates
Trader Joe's® Organic Fruit Leather	1 piece	12 carbohydrates
Jelly Belly® Jelly Beans	You choose!	1 carbohydrate per bean
Glucose tablets	1 tablet	4 carbohydrates
Restaurant sugar packet	1 packet	4 carbohydrates

Once blood sugar levels are at or fast-approaching target range again, you may want to follow up that fast-acting carb treatment. A snack with a carb + protein combo (approximately 15-20g of carbs) will help to even out the rollercoaster. Snack options for a solid blood sugar line:

Snack*

Crackers and peanut butter

Cheese and crackers

Chocolate milk

Granola bar

Trail mix

Hummus and veggies

*Look to the nutrition information for your specific snack items, as serving size and ingredients may vary.

If you are in charge of meals or snacks for the T1D in your care, you may be wondering what he or she can eat. The quick answer is that T1Ds *can* eat anything. The primary considerations that go along with food choice for someone with type 1 diabetes include that carbohydrates are accounted for and he/she is given the appropriate amount of insulin for the serving of carbs consumed. When making pre-meal insulin dose decisions, consideration should also be given to whether any amount of corrective insulin dose is necessary due to blood glucose testing results prior to the meal or snack.

That being said, the parents or doctor may have a specific eating plan or guidelines that work best for the child. Some families try to eat low-carb or limit the amount of carbs consumed. Other families keep their children on what would be recognizable as a "normal" diet for a child and simply monitor carb intake, dosing insulin accordingly. In either case, families may dose half of the insulin at the beginning of the meal, and the other half after to ensure that the child eats enough carbohydrates to prevent a low blood sugar reaction, since children can be picky or stubborn about eating/not eating. Sometimes the insulin may be given a few minutes in advance of the meal (known as "pre-bolusing") to help blunt post-meal spikes.

As long as you understand the directions for insulin dosing as given by the parents and/or medical team and follow them accordingly, you are doing everything in your power to handle food-related diabetes concerns. Count the carbohydrates and dose insulin based on the child's insulin to carb ratio, adding corrective doses as needed (based on the child's correction factor – **Chapter 3 What Causes Blood Glucose Fluctuations?**).

Carb Counting

Carbohydrates, measured in grams (g), have the most significant effect on blood sugar. Carb counting is beneficial because it allows for flexibility in diet and a targeted formula for dosing insulin. A more tailored and effective dose of insulin helps to prevent post-meal highs or lows. Reading food labels, being mindful of listed portion sizes versus actual portion consumed, utilizing measuring cups/spoons, and/or a food scale will provide the information you need to determine how many carbs are in the portion of food you are considering. The child's insulin to carb ratio (I:C) will tell you how many units of insulin need to be delivered to cover the desired amount of carbs.

Example: With an insulin to carb ratio of 1:10, a meal with 20 carbs would mean taking an insulin dose of two units.

Note: When counting carbs, take into consideration the amount of fiber in the snack or meal, as well as any sugar alcohols. There are a few ways that people do this, so consult your T1D's parents and/or medical team to determine which strategy to apply.

One common guideline indicates that for any food that contains 5 grams of fiber or more, subtract the dietary fiber from the carbohydrates before calculating the insulin dose.

Example: When eating a meal with 35 carbs and five grams of fiber, calculate 35-5=30. With a 1:10 insulin to carb ratio, the dose for that meal would be three units.

Another common guideline indicates subtracting half of the amount of the fiber present from the carbohydrates.

Example: When eating a meal with 45 carbs and 10 grams of fiber, calculate 45-5=40. With a 1:10 insulin to carb ratio, the dose for that meal would be 4 units.

If more than 5 grams of sugar alcohols are present in the food item (commonly found in sugar-free or no sugar added items), subtract half of the sugar alcohols from the carbohydrates.

For a more in-depth look at the factors in carbohydrate counting as it relates to insulin dosing and food choices, I recommend Gary Scheiner's book, *The Complete Guide to Carbohydrate Counting*.

Macronutrients

Macronutrients are nutrients that provide energy (calories). The three macronutrients are fat, protein, and carbohydrates. These macronutrients help make up the elements of a balanced meal. When taking into account meal or snack planning for optimum T1D management, think about how you choose to incorporate fat, protein, and carbohydrates.

Fat

Dietary fat is essential for important bodily progress and functions, such as brain development. There is "good" fat and "bad" fat. Good fat, also known as unsaturated fat, can be found in fish, nuts, oils (like olive oil), and avocados. Bad fat, also known as saturated fat, can be found in animal products. There is another form of bad fat, known as trans fat. We should try to eat as little trans fat as possible. Trans fat is present in processed foods, shortening, deep fried foods, margarine, and frozen food items (due to the ability of artificial trans fats to extend the shelf life of food).

Other considerations regarding fat include the consumption of Omega-3 fatty acids, which are essential to the health of the brain, eyes, and nervous system. Fish (such as salmon), vegetable oil, seed oil, and fish oils are rich in Omega-3 fatty acids.

In summary regarding dietary fats: the majority of fat consumption should be in the form of unsaturated fats and Omega-3 fatty acids, limit intake of saturated fats, and eliminate artificial trans fats whenever possible. Be aware that fat slows down the absorption of carbohydrates into the bloodstream, which may cause a delay lasting several hours in seeing a "spike" from carb consumption. Foods that may cause

58

a delay in the absorption of carbohydrates due to fat content include pizza, cheeseburgers, ice cream, etc.

Protein

Protein is utilized by the body for the growth, maintenance, and replacement of body tissue. Foods that are animal products and good sources of protein include poultry, eggs, and dairy products. Plant-based protein can be found in nuts, seeds, legumes, and grains (like quinoa). Protein will also slow down the absorption of carbohydrates in the bloodstream.

In the past, you may have heard that people with diabetes need to restrict their intake of protein. This had to do with the association between kidney-related complications to diabetes. In general, this is no longer a consideration for children with type 1 diabetes. Unless there is a specific directive issued by your T1D's health team, for this reason or another, there is no reason to be overly vigilant about protein consumption.

Carbohydrates

Carbohydrates (carbs) are processed by our bodies and made into glucose, which is then used for energy. As previously stated, people with type 1 diabetes do not have the ability to create insulin, the hormone that is responsible for processing carbohydrates into glucose for energy, which is why they need to inject or pump insulin into the body. This is why carbohydrates are the focal point for dietary considerations for people living with type 1 diabetes.

There are two types of carbohydrates: simple and complex. Simple carbohydrates are found in milk, fruit, and refined sugars, like candy or table sugar. Complex carbohydrates, or starches, are found in bread, crackers, pasta, and rice. There are healthy (and not as healthy) choices in both categories of carbohydrates. Unprocessed or minimally processed whole grains (whole oats, whole wheat, brown rice, etc.) are preferable choices to processed grains or simple carbohydrates, like white bread. Whole grain options contain fiber, which is helpful in regulating blood sugar, feeling "full" longer, and decreasing constipation. Fiber can also be found in foods such as legumes, vegetables, and some fruit.

Remember that even healthy choices such as fruit and vegetables (such as carrots and corn) will have carbs that need to be accounted for with insulin. Other meal options, like take out food or dishes that are prepared with starch, sauce, glaze, or kid favorites, like barbeque sauce and ketchup, may contain "hidden" carbs which will need to be kept in mind when dosing for a meal or snack. Check in with your T1D's parents to see how their medical team has advised them to handle bolusing for condiments.

Putting It All Together

How might you consider combining the three macronutrients (fat, protein, and carbohydrates) for a balanced meal with a good chance of in-range post-meal blood glucose numbers? Here are some things to think about:

Every body is different. There are so many factors to consider when developing an ideal meal for a child with T1D. Food allergies, caloric intake for weight management, the amount of physical activity undertaken by the T1D, and general level of pickiness can all be considerations when determining meal or snack content, not to mention the desire for in-range glycemic control/in-range blood glucose levels.

Do the best you can to address these considerations. Do not let yourself be paralyzed by food fear. Remember, the child must eat the amount of carbs he/she took insulin for, regardless of whether those carbs are delivered by the meal you planned to serve or a few sips of juice at the end of the meal when the child has refused to finish eating.

Additional Considerations

Glycemic Index

Some people find that the glycemic index is a helpful resource. The glycemic index assigns ratings of carbohydrate-containing foods based upon how quickly those carbohydrates will convert to glucose, thus elevating blood glucose levels, on a scale of 1-100. As you might expect after reading about the macronutrients above, high fiber foods raise blood sugar at a slower rate than low or no fiber foods. High fat foods raise blood sugar slower than low or no fat foods. Solid foods raise blood sugar at a slower rate than liquids (this comes to mind when thinking about the availability of juice or regular soda in the case of a low blood sugar episode).

Sugar-Free

Many families choose to avoid sugar-free foods, as many of those options contain artificial chemical sweeteners that may cause gastrointestinal distress. Also, despite the common misconception that someone with diabetes can eat as much sugar-free food as they want, we know that just because something is sugar-free does not mean that it is carbohydrate-free (or that it won't upset tummies). As we learned earlier in the chapter, today's standard of care for dosing insulin in individuals with type 1 diabetes is dependent upon counting carbohydrates, not sugar content, thus alleviating the need to rely on sugar-free foods.

Commonly, individuals and families choose carefully which sugar-free items they are willing to consume, and which they will avoid. For example, I have made a decision for myself that I would rather eat a smaller amount of a delicious, carb-rich meal or dessert than a sugar-free substitute that would make me feel like I was still missing out on the food I wanted to eat. I actively avoid any sugar-free candy or baked goods and do not use any sugar substitutes when I cook or bake. However, I occasionally indulge in Diet Coke® (sugar-free, carb-free) or sugar-free gelatin (easy snack with a very small amount of artificial sweetener). That is my personal preference and what I feel works best for me.

Ask your T1D's family what they and their medical team have determined is best regarding choosing or avoiding sugar-free items.

T1D + Celiac Disease

A common co-condition to type 1 diabetes is celiac disease, an immune reaction to eating gluten, a protein found in wheat, barley, and rye. If this, or another form of gluten sensitivity, is something your T1D is dealing with, you will quickly become familiar with what meal and snack choices work best to avoid gluten reactions and stay within treatment guidelines for diabetes as well.

Common foods that you will come across that often contain gluten include:

- pasta/noodles

- breads/pastries

- crackers

- cereals/granola

- flour tortillas

Also, gluten is sometimes "hidden" in foods and things you might not think of as containing gluten, such as sauces and soups (flour as thickening agent), salad dressings, marinades, soy sauce, or even non-ingestible items like lip balm or play dough. Some tablet medications also contain gluten, via wheat starch that acts as a binder for the tablet. Even communion wafers are likely to contain gluten, so be aware. The best way to know if something has gluten is to verify.

Look for certified gluten-free labeling on packaged items and ingredients and do not be afraid to ask at restaurants about whether menu selections are gluten-free and/or have the potential for cross-contamination on a grill, in a fryer, etc. If you are unable to verify the validity of the gluten-free status, you will want to pass on that item and look for a gluten-free alternative.

CHAPTER 8:
HYPOGLYCEMIA/LOW BLOOD SUGAR

- Low blood sugar is to be treated as an emergency

- It is the most dangerous event that can occur in the short-term in life with type 1 diabetes

- Fast-acting carbohydrates such as juice, regular soda, and candy are the treatment for low blood sugar

- Do NOT administer insulin to "treat" low blood sugar; administering insulin to treat low blood sugar is incorrect and potentially fatal, as insulin will lower blood sugar further

- Failure to treat hypoglycemia/low blood sugar can lead to seizures, coma, or death

- Keeping a close eye on blood sugar, especially during and after physical activity, will help in anticipating the situation before it becomes an emergency

- Do NOT allow a child who is low to walk anywhere alone, including the school health office

- Following a low blood sugar treatment of fast sugar with a carb + protein combo snack will help to prevent a rebound high or secondary lows

Hypoglycemia is typically defined as when a person's blood glucose level falls to 70 mg/dl and below. However, as with many aspects of diabetes, the threshold at which attention needs to be paid to dropping blood sugar levels (and at what number to begin treating to raise BG levels) may occur at a different number per parental or medical order.

The symptoms of hypoglycemia are:

- Shakiness

- Dizziness

- Confusion

- Nausea

- Headache

- Slurred speech

- Impaired coordination

You might hear someone refer to hypoglycemia as "low blood glucose," "low blood sugar," or even just simply a "hypo" or "low." It does not matter what you call it, as long as you know how to recognize and treat it when it occurs. When caring for a child with diabetes, it is important to note that what constitutes a low or a blood glucose level requiring further attention or treatment may be a higher number than 70, so **be sure to check with the parents and medical care plan to be informed about the target range for your T1D.**

Depending on the age and/or communication skills of the child, he or she may be unable to directly and efficiently notify you when they are experiencing low blood sugar. Even adults who have lived with the disease for decades sometimes struggle to recognize or seek assistance when experiencing a low. You may notice unusual behavior before the T1D does, like stumbling, trouble speaking, or anything that just does not seem right. Whether you catch the behavior or he/she expresses feeling unwell, the first step is to whip out the glucometer and check blood glucose levels (see **Chapter 4 – How to Use a Glucose Meter** for a refresher on this process). You want to quickly confirm that the child is experiencing symptoms as a result of low blood sugar and not because of something else, such as a concussion.

Do NOT allow a child who is experiencing low blood sugar or expressing symptoms of low blood sugar to walk anywhere alone. Not to the bathroom, not to the health office, not to their house next door. If you must send the child somewhere, they must be accompanied by a buddy who can call for help, if needed. Better yet, handle the treatment of the low blood glucose levels in place, where the T1D can be safely supervised until they are feeling better.

If you have access to a CGM (See **Chapter 6-How to Use a Continuous Glucose Monitor**), you may be able to spot a falling pattern over time or see that glucose levels are taking a dive, enabling you to pull out the meter kit before levels land in dangerous territory. If the number on the meter is low or close to low range with a CGM reading that indicates an imminent fall, prepare to treat hypoglycemia. It is a wonderful and important tool, but remember that CGM is not a replacement for vigilance by the T1D and caregiver or verification by checking with a meter.

Treating Hypoglycemia/Low Blood Sugar

How to treat hypoglycemia? Great question, and an exceptionally important one at that. **The treatment for low blood sugar is fast-acting carbohydrates (simple sugars).**

There's a rule of 15 that many diabetes clinics recommend; give 15 grams of fast-acting carbohydrates and wait 15 minutes to check the status of BG before giving another 15 grams of carbohydrate until reaching the target number. This rule is more of a guideline. This is another important thing to check on in the child's care plan, as their parent or doctor may have a more tailored treatment directive. However, when in doubt, treat the low. If you overshoot with the fast-acting carbs, it can be corrected later. Hypoglycemia is dangerous in the moment. If left untreated, it can lead to seizures, coma, or death. I do not want to scare you with that information, but simply impress upon you how important treating this issue is for a person with diabetes. When in doubt (about BG number, how much fast-acting carbohydrate to use, how long to wait between checking BG, etc.), give fast-acting carbs and correct with insulin later, if needed.

Examples of fast-acting carbohydrates for the treatment of hypoglycemia:

- Fruit juice

- Regular soda

- Glucose tablets/gels (available at your local pharmacy)

- Candy (go for dextrose-based items, if possible, while avoiding chocolate [the fat in chocolate slows down the absorption of the carbohydrates into the bloodstream, which delays the elevation of blood glucose levels])

- Sugar cubes/packets (conveniently portioned into 4 carbohydrate units)

Hypoglycemia can affect behavior, motor skills, attitude, and critical thinking abilities. Please remember to check blood glucose when these unusual disruptions occur instead of first assuming there is an attitude problem on the part of the child. **When hypoglycemia occurs, it is an immediate issue that requires immediate attention.** Do not make the child complete an activity or wait until you have a free moment to address the issue. By the time this happens, what could have been an easily treated mild low could become a severe situation that requires emergency services. Hypoglycemia is an easily treated issue that comes up in life with T1D; emergencies are rare, but possible, and are often a result of failing to recognize or treat the situation when it first arises.

If blood glucose levels continue to lower rapidly, despite continued treatment, contact your T1D's parents (again, consult the individual care plan for detailed wishes and instructions). If the situation is deteriorating and/or you feel it is no longer something that you can safely and confidently handle in the current setting, do not hesitate to call 911. The dispatcher may walk you through the administration of a Glucagon emergency kit, which we will be discussing in the next chapter.

CHAPTER 9:
IN CASE OF EMERGENCY:
ADMINISTERING GLUCAGON

- Seek instructions and training for Glucagon use from a certified medical professional

- In the case of hypoglycemia (low blood sugar) that results in a combative or unresponsive person with diabetes, using a Glucagon kit is the next step of treatment

- Be sure to know where your T1D's Glucagon kit is kept and know how to use it

- If the T1D in your care is seizing, combative, unresponsive, or unconscious, call 911 immediately

Glucagon is the hormone released by the liver to keep blood sugar up and even, acting as a counterpart to insulin. In a non-diabetic person, the liver produces and utilizes glucagon automatically. Glucagon sets in motion the process of liver and muscle modifying glycogen into glucose in order to release glucose back into your bloodstream, keeping blood glucose levels from dropping or staying dangerously low.

A Glucagon emergency kit is an item that should be kept on hand for extreme hypoglycemic emergencies. In general, administering Glucagon for the treatment of low blood sugar is rare, as addressing low blood sugar immediately when it first occurs often is an effective preventative measure to avoid Glucagon emergency treatment. Typically, situations that necessitate the use of a Glucagon emergency kit are marked by the person with diabetes experiencing severe hypoglycemia (low blood sugar) resulting in seizure, loss of consciousness, or combative behavior. In other cases, the child with diabetes may be prone to rapidly changing blood glucose levels.

Currently, both Eli Lilly and Company and Novo Nordisk® manufacture hypoglycemia emergency kits. Eli Lilly's is known by the name Glucagon (red plastic case) and Novo Nordisk's is called GlucaGen® HypoKit® (orange plastic case). Each kit will have instructions inside, but it is important to familiarize yourself with the process of mixing and administering in advance. If possible, you may also consider downloading the Glucagon by Eli Lilly and Company app in your mobile phone application store to have on hand in case of an emergency, since it can walk you through the process. Becoming familiar with the mixing instructions and administration process ahead of time will assure that no time is wasted if presented with an emergency situation.

If you were to encounter a situation where administering Glucagon was necessary, you would want to call 911. If you have questions about this, or feel unclear about whether or not you would call 911 when administering Glucagon, discuss with the child's parents and/or medical team.

Be sure to dispose of unused Glucagon. Once mixed, any unused Glucagon can be kept in the refrigerator for up to 24 hours. After this point, the mixture will no longer be effective. Also, dispose of any sharps appropriately after use.

We all hope that knowing how to administer Glucagon is a skill that we will never need to use. By being prepared with the knowledge and skill to do so, we mitigate the possibility of being confronted with a scary and dangerous situation that cannot be handled successfully. Knowing how to handle the situation will build your confidence and ability, should you ever be faced with a moment where it is necessary.

Panic can cause us to rush or forget an important step. Do not forget that the powder and saline must be mixed in the vial before being drawn back out for delivery by syringe. Omitting this step and delivering saline solution alone is a mistake that could be deadly. If you are knowledgeable and prepared, you are unlikely to make this error.

Being knowledgeable and prepared, you will snap right into action and handle business straightaway, delivering the child from the serious complications of extreme low blood sugar. Later, you can high-five each other for making it through.

Keep expired Glucagon kits and mark them "expired." Replace them with the new kit wherever you have kept them in the past. Be sure to let all caregiving parties know if you change the location of the Glucagon kit(s). Use the expired Glucagon kits to practice mixing and administering so you will feel more comfortable in the situation of having to take out the Glucagon in an emergency situation. If you are in need of further practice with Glucagon, the pharmaceutical company Eli Lilly has practice kits that can be requested. Knowledge (and experience) is power!

In case of extreme low blood sugar resulting in the inability to swallow, seizures, physical aggression, or unconsciousness, **administer a Glucagon emergency kit**

(red or orange plastic box), as directed by the T1D diabetes management plan and medical team.

The **Quick Reference** section provides step-by-step instructions for Glucagon administration for quick access. Here is the complete information for the user, reprinted with permission from Eli Lilly and Company for your safety and convenience:

INFORMATION FOR THE USER

GLUCAGON FOR INJECTION (rDNA ORIGIN)

BECOME FAMILIAR WITH THE FOLLOWING INSTRUCTIONS BEFORE AN EMERGENCY ARISES. DO NOT USE THIS KIT AFTER DATE STAMPED ON THE BOTTLE LABEL. IF YOU HAVE QUESTIONS CONCERNING THE USE OF THIS PRODUCT, CONSULT A DOCTOR, NURSE OR PHARMACIST.

Make sure that your relatives or close friends know that if you become unconscious, medical assistance must always be sought. Glucagon may have been prescribed so that members of your household can give the injection if you become hypoglycemic and are unable to take sugar by mouth. If you are unconscious, Glucagon can be given while awaiting medical assistance.

Show your family members and others where you keep this kit and how to use it. They need to know how to use it before you need it. They can practice giving a shot by giving you your normal insulin shots. It is important that they practice. A person who has never given a shot probably will not be able to do it in an emergency.

IMPORTANT

- Act quickly. Prolonged unconsciousness may be harmful.
- These simple instructions will help you give Glucagon successfully.
- Turn patient on his/her side to prevent patient from choking.
- The contents of the syringe are inactive. You must mix the contents of the syringe with the Glucagon in the accompanying bottle before giving injection. (*See* DIRECTIONS FOR USE below.)

Do not prepare Glucagon for Injection until you are ready to use it.

WARNING: THE PATIENT MAY BE IN A COMA FROM SEVERE HYPERGLYCEMIA (HIGH BLOOD GLUCOSE) RATHER THAN HYPOGLYCEMIA. IN SUCH A CASE, THE PATIENT WILL **NOT** RESPOND TO GLUCAGON AND REQUIRES IMMEDIATE MEDICAL ATTENTION.

INDICATIONS FOR USE

Use Glucagon to treat insulin coma or insulin reaction resulting from severe hypoglycemia (low blood sugar). Symptoms of severe hypoglycemia include disorientation, unconsciousness, and seizures or convulsions. Give Glucagon if
(1) the patient is unconscious
(2) the patient is unable to eat sugar or a sugar-sweetened product
(3) the patient is having a seizure, or
(4) repeated administration of sugar or a sugar-sweetened product such as a regular soft drink or fruit juice does not improve the patient's condition. Milder cases of hypoglycemia should be treated promptly by eating sugar or a sugar-sweetened product.
(*See* INFORMATION ON HYPOGLYCEMIA below for more information on the symptoms of hypoglycemia.)
Glucagon is not active when taken orally.

DIRECTIONS FOR USE

TO PREPARE GLUCAGON FOR INJECTION

1. Remove the flip-off seal from the bottle of Glucagon. Wipe rubber stopper on bottle with alcohol swab.

2. Remove the needle protector from the syringe, and inject the entire contents of the syringe into the bottle of Glucagon. DO NOT REMOVE THE PLASTIC CLIP FROM THE SYRINGE. Remove syringe from the bottle.
3. Swirl bottle gently until Glucagon dissolves completely. GLUCAGON SHOULD NOT BE USED UNLESS THE SOLUTION IS CLEAR AND OF A WATER-LIKE CONSISTENCY.

TO INJECT GLUCAGON
Use Same Technique as for Injecting Insulin
4. Using the same syringe, hold bottle upside down and, making sure the needle tip remains in solution, gently withdraw all of the solution (1 mg mark on syringe) from bottle. The plastic clip on the syringe will prevent the rubber stopper from being pulled out of the syringe; however, if the plastic plunger rod separates from the rubber stopper, simply reinsert the rod by turning it clockwise.

The usual adult dose is 1 mg (1 unit). For children weighing less than 44 lb (20 kg), give 1/2 adult dose (0.5 mg). For children, withdraw 1/2 of the solution from the bottle (0.5 mg mark on syringe). DISCARD UNUSED PORTION.

USING THE FOLLOWING DIRECTIONS, INJECT GLUCAGON IMMEDIATELY AFTER MIXING.
5. Cleanse injection site on buttock, arm, or thigh with alcohol swab.

6. Insert the needle into the loose tissue under the cleansed injection site, and inject all (or 1/2 for children weighing less than 44 lb) of the Glucagon solution. THERE IS NO DANGER OF OVERDOSE. Apply light pressure at the injection site, and withdraw the needle. Press an alcohol swab against the injection site.

7. Turn the patient on his/her side. When an unconscious person awakens, he/she may vomit. Turning the patient on his/her side will prevent him/her from choking.

8. FEED THE PATIENT AS SOON AS HE/SHE AWAKENS AND IS ABLE TO SWALLOW. Give the patient a fast-acting source of sugar (such as a regular soft drink or fruit juice) and a long-acting source of sugar (such as crackers and cheese or a meat sandwich). If the patient does not awaken within 15 minutes, give another dose of Glucagon and INFORM A DOCTOR OR EMERGENCY SERVICES IMMEDIATELY.

9. Even if the Glucagon revives the patient, his/her doctor should be promptly notified. A doctor should be notified whenever severe hypoglycemic reactions occur.

INFORMATION ON HYPOGLYCEMIA

Early symptoms of hypoglycemia (low blood glucose) include:

- sweating
- dizziness
- palpitation
- tremor
- hunger
- restlessness
- tingling in the hands, feet, lips, or tongue
- lightheadedness
- inability to concentrate
- headache
- drowsiness
- sleep disturbances
- anxiety
- blurred vision
- slurred speech
- depressed mood
- irritability
- abnormal behavior
- unsteady movement
- personality changes

If not treated, the patient may progress to severe hypoglycemia that can include:

• disorientation
• seizures
• unconsciousness
• death

The occurrence of early symptoms calls for prompt and, if necessary, repeated administration of some form of carbohydrate. Patients should always carry a quick source of sugar, such as candy, mints or glucose tablets. The prompt treatment of mild hypoglycemic symptoms can prevent severe hypoglycemic reactions. If the patient does not improve or if administration of carbohydrate is impossible, Glucagon should be given or the patient should be treated with intravenous glucose at a medical facility. Glucagon, a naturally occurring substance produced by the pancreas, is helpful because it enables the patient to produce his/her own blood glucose to correct the hypoglycemia.

POSSIBLE PROBLEMS WITH GLUCAGON TREATMENT
Severe side effects are very rare, although nausea and vomiting may occur occasionally.
A few people may be allergic to Glucagon or to one of the inactive ingredients in Glucagon, or may experience rapid heart beat for a short while.
If you experience any other reactions which are likely to have been caused by Glucagon, please contact your doctor.

STORAGE
Before dissolving Glucagon with diluting solution — Store the kit at controlled room temperature between 20° to 25°C (68° to 77°F).
After dissolving Glucagon with diluting solution — Should be used immediately. **Discard any unused portion.** Solutions should be clear and of a water-like consistency at time of use.

Please consult the manufacturer direction insert, parents, and/or medical team, for detailed instruction regarding the administration of Glucagon. The information published here is for general knowledge and is not meant to be clinical in nature.

Literature revised September 19, 2012
Marketed by: Lilly USA, LLC Indianapolis, IN 46285, USA
PA 2286 AMP

CHAPTER 10:
HYPERGLYCEMIA/HIGH BLOOD SUGAR

- Sustained elevated blood sugar levels will cause discomfort in the short-term and the complications we seek to avoid in the long-term

- High blood sugar is sometimes accompanied by ketones, which can be measured with blood ketone meters or urine keto strips

- Diabetic ketoacidosis (DKA) is a serious complication of high blood sugar that necessitates immediate emergency medical attention

Hyperglycemia is defined as a blood glucose level of 180-250 mg/dl and above, although each T1D has a different threshold for concern. Check with the parents and/or medical team to find out at what number to begin treating high blood sugar when the child is in your care.

The signs of hyperglycemia (or elevated blood glucose levels) include:

- Frequent urination

- Increased thirst

- Trouble concentrating

- Blurred vision

- Irritability

- Headache

Some people might ask, "If low blood sugar episodes (hypoglycemia) are so dangerous in the short term, why not run a person's blood sugar at a higher number so as not to risk a hypo?"

The short answer is that while low blood sugar is indeed dangerous in the short term, chronic elevated blood glucose levels will not only cause a person to feel sluggish or ill, but will also increase the likelihood of complications due to diabetes in the long-term.

What are Ketones?

Ketones are the result of the body burning fat for energy in place of carbohydrates/glucose. In the absence of adequate insulin, the body is unable to process the glucose present in the bloodstream and begins to break down fat for energy instead. If left untreated, this can lead to a life-threatening complication of type 1 diabetes called diabetic ketoacidosis.

Checking for Ketones

There are two ways to test for ketones: urinalysis strips (easily purchased over the counter at the pharmacy in a pinch) or blood ketone meter. A general recommendation is to test for ketones when a fingerstick blood test shows results of 250 mg/dl or higher.

This is a topic that truly needs to be discussed with the T1D parents and/or medical team, as some children are more prone to ketones or developing diabetic ketoacidosis (DKA) than others, which may mean a more aggressive plan of treatment or visit to the emergency room.

Consult with your T1D's parents and/or medical team to determine what their process is for identifying and treating ketones.

Diabetic Ketoacidosis

Diabetic ketoacidosis is a serious complication of hyperglycemia that occurs when a lack of insulin causes glucose to build up in the blood. When cells are unable to use glucose for energy, the body burns fat and muscle instead. This causes ketones to appear in the bloodstream, creating a dangerous metabolic imbalance that will eventually shut down the body if left untreated.

If the child wears an insulin pump and is experiencing hyperglycemia and/or tests positive for ketones, check to make sure the pump is delivering insulin. If there is an occlusion (blockage) in the tubing, kink in the cannula, or any other sort of malfunction, insulin delivery will cease, causing elevated glucose levels, ketones, and, if left untreated, diabetic ketoacidosis.

The symptoms of diabetic ketoacidosis (DKA) are:

- confusion
- blurred vision
- physical weakness
- rapid breathing
- fruity/acetone scent on breath (the odor of ketones)
- dry mouth
- nausea or vomiting
- abdominal pain
- loss of appetite

- fatigue

- excessive thirst

- dehydration

- weight loss

If the child in your care is presenting with the symptoms of DKA, treat this as an immediate emergency situation. Take the child to an emergency room. Call ahead, if possible, letting them know that you are bringing a child with type 1 diabetes who is exhibiting the symptoms of DKA. They will prepare for your arrival. If the child is already unconscious, call an ambulance.

Section 3:
Caregiver Confidence

CHAPTER 11:
SOLUTIONS FOR SPECIAL OCCASIONS

Classroom/Daycare/Camp Celebrations, Birthday Parties, Field Trips and Travel

- Kids are kids first. They are kids living with type 1 diabetes second

- Special occasions do not have to occur differently for children with diabetes

- Forethought and preparation will help make things run smoothly for all involved

Life happens while we are living it. This means that diabetes does not occur in a vacuum, but while we are encountering things like festivities in the classroom, birthday parties, field trips, or travel with friends/family. We strive to build environments where remarkable experiences and memories develop naturally, with a little extra thought and preparation for safety and well-being. By finding creative solutions for participating in life's special occasions, we lighten the burden of diabetes from the small shoulders of these children for whom we care so deeply.

Here are some common concerns and considerations for parents and caregivers in what can feel like difficult circumstances, along with solutions to build both the child's and your confidence in dealing with T1D out in the world.

Classroom/Daycare/Camp Celebrations

When birthdays or other celebrations approach, it almost certainly means there will be sweet treats and carbohydrate-rich snacks to follow. Unless specific instructions from the child's parents and/or medical team state otherwise, assume that the child can and will participate in the celebration. A few ways that parents and schools can work together to make this a seamless experience for everyone involved include:

- Agreeing to communicate via text with the child's parents when treats or food comes into the classroom/daycare/camp. Taking a quick picture to send to the parent to visually estimate a carb count for insulin dosing is good for keeping everybody in the loop and avoiding miscommunications.

- Communicating ahead of time regarding when the food will be served can help eliminate an extra injection for children on MDI. For example, if the treat is served at lunchtime, the nurse (or whoever is overseeing insulin delivery) can add the appropriate amount to the dose already scheduled.

- A strategy that is successful for parents who feel more comfortable knowing exactly what their child is eating (particularly if they are dealing with food allergies and/or celiac in addition to T1D): sending in homemade treats to keep in the office freezer to take out when celebrations occur. Since the parent is preparing the items, they will be able to provide the exact carb count, as well as know that their child will not be at risk of eating an ingredient that will have a negative effect upon their well-being or cause an allergic reaction.

Invite parents to be an active participant in the planning of these special events. If they are available, they may be interested in volunteering to help, which would also enable them to oversee the handling of treats until there is a level of familiarity and comfort for everyone involved.

Birthday Parties

Everyone loves a good party! Having a child with type 1 diabetes in attendance does not have to change anything. As always, consult with the parents to confirm that they are on board with this approach, but recommendations or requests for parties are commonly aligned with what you likely would have chosen to do, regardless.

- As the host, provide activities that do not center on food. Games, crafts, or other fun keeps the emphasis off of excessive consumption of carbohydrates for everyone.

- Offer low-carb or carb-free food and drink options for all of your guests. Many guests will appreciate these types of menu options, including type 1 families. Think about putting water bottles (and maybe a sugar-free drink option, like diet soda or Crystal Light® lemonade) out with the soda. Place a platter of veggies and dip as an alternative to chips.

- Speaking with the parents beforehand helps to eliminate uncomfortable moments during the party. No need to ostracize or put the child on the spot with an awkward "You can't eat that, right?"

- When it comes to cutting the cake, proceed normally. Unless the parent has communicated with you that their child should not be given a piece of cake, go ahead and serve a reasonably-sized portion and ensure that the child remembers to bolus for the treat.

- Keep in mind that birthday fun like bounce houses or active games can cause a dip in blood sugar. Monitor levels closely. You can use the birthday sweets as a treatment for low blood sugar, if needed.

- Any information you might have regarding the carb count in the foods served at the party will help for insulin dosing purposes. Whether it means holding off on throwing away packaging or having an idea of the ingredient list and quantity in homemade items, that information will be helpful and greatly appreciated when it comes time to bolus and eat.

- Parties that include an overnight component will require communication between the T1D's parents and host parents regarding insulin dosing needs, preparation for low blood sugar, and how to use relevant diabetes devices, including a blood glucose meter. The plan will vary depending on the age of the partygoer, as well as the comfort and knowledge level of the host family. Everyone approaches slumber parties a little bit differently and whatever approach works best to provide for health, safety, and fun for each unique situation is the way to go.

Field Trips

Students with T1D should not face barriers in attending field trips with their peers. This is a highly individualized area and may vary depending upon the length and location of the field trip, as well as written modifications in 504 plans, individualized education plans (IEPs), individualized health plans (IHPs), diabetes medical management plans (DMMPs), and the local laws and requirements governing schools in your area. These are just a few things to keep in mind to help you determine your field trip plan.

The following topics can help spark conversation when discussing the situation of your T1D with their parents or medical team.

- Advance preparation is key for a calm and enjoyable field trip experience. A field trip schedule distributed to parents at the beginning of the school year can help facilitate planning ahead and mitigate last minute issues. This allows time for communication, training, or addressing any concerns when putting a field trip plan in place.

- Regardless of whether it is the parent, a school-provided nurse, or other volunteer, there always needs to be an individual trained in how to care for the child and manage T1D on the trip.

- Supplies and back up materials must make it onto the bus with the student and their T1D field trip caregiver. Once the bus has arrived at the destination, the supplies must accompany the student throughout the trip. Supplies must be accessible and convenient for diabetes management at all times during the trip. Depending on the age of the student, these items may either be carried by the student or the adult assigned to T1D care. The care routine remains just as important when away from home and school as it is normally.

Travel

Going somewhere? Take a few minutes to prepare for your trip with your T1D and you will be ready to enjoy the sights and sounds of your destination when you arrive. Consult with the parents and medical team regarding specifics for the individual child. Here are a few things to consider when preparing for a fun trip with your T1D.

- Make a list of supplies. Check it twice. Carry copies of prescriptions and ratios, contact information for supply manufacturers (in case of device failure). You will want to have extras of everything, including pump supplies, insulin, and low treatments. Carry supplies in two different bags, in case one bag gets lost or stolen.

- Bring a note from the doctor regarding the necessity of traveling with syringes, juice, etc.

- If you are traveling by plane, give your group extra time to get through security. Manufacturers of diabetes drugs and supplies have recommendations regarding whether their products can go through x-ray machines and/or body scanners. Keeping all of your supplies together can help expedite the security process by allowing you to pull it out for inspection while putting the rest of your travel gear through the machines. Consider keeping solid low treatments instead of liquids (such as glucose tablets or candy instead of juice) to more easily get through the security process. Do not put supplies in checked bags!

- Also for plane travel: some individuals, particularly pump users, report "baggage claim lows" after arriving at their destination (experiencing low blood sugar after disembarking an airplane, around the time one would be grabbing luggage off the carousel or leaving the airport). Being prepared with travel snacks will help you get through any baggage claim lows on your way to the next stop.

- The climate at your destination may necessitate that insulin and/or other supplies will need to be kept in a temperature-controlled container (cooler, cooling wallet, etc.). Remember to make these arrangements in advance, as insulin that has been exposed to extreme heat or cold will no longer be effective.

- If you plan to keep insulin in a hotel refrigerator, confirm that your room will have a refrigerator prior to your arrival— also be aware that hotel refrigerator temperatures are nearly impossible to control, so you may be better off using your own guaranteed method of stored temperature control or leaving it at room temperature if the climate allows. You must ensure that the temperature setting will not cause the insulin to freeze, as frozen insulin, even once thawed, will **not** work and you will need an emergency replacement.

- Remember, climate and altitude can also have an effect on blood sugar levels.

- Stay consistent with the diabetes care routine, as much as possible. Travel brings excitement, stress, and unexpected ups and downs. Being prepared and staying consistent with care are your two best tools for an easy and fun travel experience.

Have a great trip!

CHAPTER 12:
COMMUNICATING ABOUT DIABETES

- Misinformation and stigma around diabetes means that people often, knowingly or unknowingly, say things to or about people with type 1 that can cause perpetuated false stereotypes or hurt a child's feelings

- Taking into account tone and an individual's preference toward people-first language (person with diabetes) or identity-first language (diabetic) is one way to consider how we communicate about this disease

The words we use have meaning and the words we use to communicate about diabetes are no different. Words and phrases that come from a place of positivity, encouragement, and respect create an environment for success and empowerment. Words and phrases that treat a T1D with negativity, ridicule, and shame (whether knowingly or unknowingly) can make a huge impact on emotional health. In cases when we communicate about diabetes to people who live unaffected by diabetes, it is important to have a grasp on the definition of the disease and how to speak about it because we lead by example. Many times, people who say demeaning things about diabetes or people with diabetes do not realize that what they are saying is false and/or hurtful. It is up to us, people who love and care about people who live with this burdensome disease, to kindly and firmly educate while presenting ourselves as role models in how to advocate for others.

Tone

The tone we use when speaking about diabetes (especially when we speak to, or in front of, children) can carry more meaning than the actual words coming out of our mouths. When dealing with a child, it is easy to slip into an accusatory tone. Be mindful that if you are displaying your frustration or irritation with the disease, the child might interpret that as frustration or irritation with them or something they did or did not do. When you recognize yourself making these feelings known, take a breather. Tell the child that your frustration or irritation is with the disease or whatever element that is bothering you in that moment. Let them know that they are not the cause of the problem. If the child did do something that is related to the cause of the issue, consider waiting until your anger has passed so that you can have a calm, interactive exchange about what went wrong and what can be done to avoid that issue in the future. When these moments occur, use them as a learning tool to help prevent these issues going forward.

People-First Language or Identity-First Language

Just like diabetes management, diabetes language and mindset are individual as well. The way we choose to describe ourselves is personal and contributes to how we approach our condition, our relationships, and ourselves with others in this context. Being open to conversation about changing preferences or feelings that come up when being addressed as a person with diabetes (PWD), diabetic, or otherwise, will be important.

The people-first language movement is about seeing an individual as a person first and patient second, as patients should not be defined by their diagnoses. To some children and families, this distinction is extremely important. You will not find these individuals referring to their T1D as "diabetic" or "a diabetic." If this is their preference, please respect it and encourage others to do so as well. The people-first way to refer to someone with diabetes is "person with diabetes" or PWD, for short.

The identity-first language movement chooses to see the identity of the individual as involving his/her condition. Some individuals feel strongly that people-first language robs them of a large part of their identity; stripping them of a descriptor that helps explain who they are and what their life's story entails. Individuals who prefer identity-first language might refer to themselves as (a) diabetic. If this is their preference, please respect it and encourage others to do so as well.

There are also people who may not have a strong preference as to the language used. Some are fine with any accurate descriptor, and that is their prerogative. Personally, I find it more expedient in certain conversations to say that I am diabetic or a type 1 diabetic just to get the message across more quickly.

I have also been known to say I "live with type 1 diabetes" or simply that I "have" type 1. I resist feeling offended by the descriptor "diabetic," so long as it is not being used in a truly pejorative manner. I have friends who feel differently about the topic, so I am sure to respect their feelings and wishes regarding people-first language when we are together.

Other communication-related topics that make a difference in the mindset of many people living with T1D is the choice in how we present certain common phrases in order to come from a place of patient empowerment, being the experts in our own condition and bodies. Certain ways of phrasing diabetes tasks encourage a positive emphasis on the process of taking care of

T1D, instead of focusing on the outcome, which can become negative.

Here are a few examples, listed with their preferred alternatives:

Common Phrases	Preferred Alternatives
(non) compliance /compliant	(non) adherence/adherent
control	management
control	in-range
diabetic	person with diabetes
test	check
suffering from	living with

CHAPTER 13:
EMOTIONS OF DIABETES

- Type 1 diabetes is as much an invisible illness as it is a physical one

- People with T1D usually appear to "look healthy"

- Much of the time T1Ds appear happy and unburdened by this disease (but things are not always as they seem)

- We hope to build strength and resilience in our T1Ds, but it is still a difficult condition to process, especially when combined with the regular childhood/teen desire to fit in

An aspect of diabetes that someone who is unaffected by the disease may never see is the psychological and psychosocial effects of the illness. Children with type 1 diabetes are more likely to experience depression and/or anxiety than the general population. Common emotions reported by people living with T1D include fear, shame, guilt, anxiety, and sadness for the individual with T1D, as well as their family and caregivers.

Bullying/Exclusion

Children sometimes face issues with inclusion due to other children (and sometimes even adults) fearing or mocking the unknown of diabetes. If there is bullying happening at school, teachers may consider planning a lesson around type 1 diabetes to eliminate ignorance about what the disease is, how it affects your T1D, and encouraging students to be a friend and ally instead of foe. Keep parents aware of any diabetes-related issues in the classroom and invite them to present to the class or intervene, if appropriate.

Identifying Diabetes Burnout

Type 1 diabetes is a disease that requires much from the person living with it. There are non-stop evaluations and decisions being made regarding care 24 hours a day, 7 days a week, 365 days a year. The physical and emotional burden of T1D can cause periods of diabetes burnout. High levels of stress, anxiety, and sadness relating to diabetes can be indicators of burnout. Children and teens with type 1 diabetes are more susceptible to anxiety, depression, and eating disorders. If you observe behavior that is symptomatic of a serious mental health condition, get them help as quickly as possible.

If you observe the T1D in your life acting out or withdrawing related to their care regimen, concerns about the disease in their life, or how they are being treated by their peers, please address this with their family and/or medical team in order to get them the help that they need to overcome this period of challenge. There are social workers and psychologists who can provide counseling or therapy to treat these diabetes-specific issues. Listening, providing support, and rallying around families with T1D when distress or burnout comes up can help those affected to know that they are not alone.

Resources for Knowledge and Support

You do not have to tackle the complexities of this illness all on your own. There are many places for you to seek out knowledge and support for yourself and your T1D.

Non-Profit Organizations

JDRF, formerly known as the Juvenile Diabetes Research Foundation, is the leading organization funding type 1 diabetes (T1D) research for a cure and improved quality of life in the meanwhile. Online articles and sources of information are available on their website, jdrf.org, and social media. There are local chapters that host events to connect families with others also living with type 1, as well as provide Bags of Hope and toolkits for newly diagnosed individuals and families.

American Diabetes Association (ADA) is a resource for individuals and families living with both type 1 and type 2 diabetes. The ADA website, diabetes.org, is a source of general information, as well as a place to find resources about ensuring safety at school, daycare, and camp, and general legal assistance as it relates to diabetes. The ADA has regional offices around the country.

Children with Diabetes serves as a multi-function resource. The CWD website, childrenwithdiabetes.com, maintains an extensive database of information that relates to children and families living with type 1 diabetes, as well as discussion forums and even diabetes humor. Children with Diabetes also hosts notable conferences and events across the United States, Canada, and the United Kingdom. Past attendees hail the Friends for Life annual conference in Orlando, Florida as one of the best places to learn about T1D and meet families and caregivers just like you.

Project Blue November was created by a group of mothers of children with type 1 diabetes in order to provide a central online location for information and resources related to T1D. Their website, projectbluenovember.com, and social media outlets have information and resources ranging from holiday carb counts to travel tips.

Beyond Type 1 provides first-person narrative stories about varying perspectives on living with T1D on their website, beyondtype1.org, as well as information that is useful for day-to-day life with diabetes and situations that come up over the lifecycle. Beyond Type 1 also has a Snail Mail Club, which is a pen pal program for kids with diabetes to connect with their peers. The resources made available by Beyond Type 1 may also be accessed via their mobile app.

Medical Professionals

Pediatric endocrinology clinics at local hospitals employ a staff of pediatric endocrinologists, nurse practitioners, certified diabetes educators (CDEs), dietitians, and social workers. These people work with children with T1D day in and day out and are a great resource for families and caregivers alike. Many of these clinics have emergency question hotlines that can be called after hours.

Allied health professionals, such as **wellness coaches and diabetes educators,** are also a resource to consult when seeking support in dealing with a new diagnosis, reaching health and wellness goals, facing challenges or seeking accountability, or in times when extra support in the management of life with diabetes is needed. It is important to find a coach who has training and certification from a recognized and well-respected program.

Diabetes Online Community (DOC)

The diabetes online community (DOC) is a vast network of people all over the world who make their voices heard via websites, blogs, podcasts, apps, and social media. The DOC is a great place to turn to for support, knowledge, real-life experience, and information regarding advocacy.

CHAPTER 14:
DIABETES IMPROV

- T1D is unique and unpredictable

- Embrace the "Yes, and..." rule of improv comedy

- Be prepared and do your best

The tricky thing about T1D (as if there were only one) is that the disease is truly unique to the individual. Even within the life and diabetes of one person, the needs, challenges, and outcomes can vary based on the hour or day. Situations can become unpredictable, quickly. We learn to come from a place of flexibility. The health, stability, and quality of life of the T1D we care for is dependent upon the way we choose to deal with the peaks and valleys that this disease will place throughout our paths.

In improvisational comedy, there is a basic rule for performance called "Yes, and..." The "Yes, and..." rule dictates that in order for the scene to continue successfully, the actor or actress must accept whatever situation has been laid out for them by their co-stars, and then add on or react to that situation based on the information given.

Caring for T1D has its own "Yes, and..." rule. There is an endless list of possible outcomes you may be presented with when caring for someone with T1D. Despite how ridiculous, unlikely, or frustrating the outcome is that you are presented with, your role is to look at it and accept it at face value. That is the "yes" part of the scenario. The "and" part comes in when you use your T1D knowledge and skill to make a decision about what to do next. T1D care is a series of these "Yes, and..." moments. Eventually some will be just as funny as actual improv comedy and others will test your patience and resolve, but you will make it through to the other side in either case.

There will be times where the directions you have been given are not working, so you will have to try something new and experiment. For every action, there is an equal and opposite reaction...but there is no guarantee that you will be able to replicate those results on another try. The management of diabetes is, as they say, an art, not a science.

The point of saying all of this is to let you know to expect an uneven playing field. Diabetes will always have the advantage, so get scrappy. Become knowledgeable. Be prepared. Mitigate risks. Be courageous. Do your best.

CHAPTER 15:
GIVE YOURSELF GRACE

- Prioritize caring for yourself, the caregiver

- You cannot "win" at diabetes, but you will do your best - that will be enough

- Be gracious to yourself in your role as caregiver

Congratulations! You have made it to the last chapter. My hope is that you are feeling confident in your abilities to care for the T1D(s) in your life. Knowledge and skills will be your foundation, but your ability to anticipate and flex your real-life experience muscle memory will get you to where you need to go.

Something you will need to keep in mind is that you are not going to be able to feel what the T1D is feeling. Depending on the age of the child, you will not be able to get verbal cues to react to or treat. What you will be able to feel is how this disease is affecting you, as a caregiver. Acknowledge those emotions and deal with them as they arise. Be sad. Get mad. Do what you have to do to clear those feelings and come back stronger.

In airplane safety, as in diabetes care, you must put on your own oxygen mask before looking after the safety of others. Give yourself time to process all of this new information, along with the responsibilities of watching after a child with type 1 diabetes. T1D does not stop, and while you are in its presence, you will not stop either. It can be a tiring and relentless routine, so figure out what you need to do to keep yourself present.

You will do the best you can. You will be prepared. You will not be perfect. Diabetes is not something you can "win" at; there is no first prize trophy. The best reward anyone can get from diabetes is seeing the one(s) we love and care for live to see another day, each day, for a lifetime, uninhibited by the challenges of this disease. You play an important role in providing the stability and normalcy in their childhood that will serve as the foundation for a bright future, without distraction or detriment from living with type 1 diabetes.

Be kind to yourself. Give yourself grace. If something goes in a way unexpected, bob and weave. Treat. Correct. But don't beat yourself up. I could tell you not to worry, but you will. At the root of that worry, though, is care. You worry because you care, and since you care, you will take to heart everything you have learned in this book and apply it to the care of your T1D, in strength and hope.

Appendix

APPENDIX A
CONFIDENT CAREGIVER GUIDE

Date:
Child(ren)'s name(s):
DOB:
Parent names:
Parent cell phone number(s):
Home address: **Cross streets:**
Home phone number:
Physician phone number:
Clinic hotline:
Pharmacy phone number:
Hospital phone number:
Parent location while out:
Phone number of parent location:

Emergency contact(s):

Times to check blood glucose (BG):

Overnight BG check schedule:

BG target range:

High BG threshold:

Usual signs of high BG:

What to do when BG is high:

Low BG threshold:

Usual signs of low BG:

What to do when BG is low:

Preferred source of fast-acting carbs and portion size:

Severe low BG threshold:

What to do if child is unresponsive:

Location of Glucagon and when to administer:

When to call 911:

List of necessary supplies and where to find them:

Basal insulin type, amount, and dose schedule:

Bolus insulin type:

Preferred injection sites:

When to administer insulin:

Insulin to carb ratio (I:C):

Correction factor:

Meal/snack times:

Food to be served:

Carb count(s):

Alternative foods if child refuses to eat:

Must-have items for outings:

Additional information:

Always call parent(s) if child has severe low blood glucose, took insulin but refuses to eat, begins to vomit, or if you have any questions on care instructions

APPENDIX B
THE CAREGIVER CONVERSATION

These are questions designed to build rapport between you, the caregiver, and the parent(s) of the T1D in your care. Starting the caregiving conversation can be daunting, but using one of the questions below as a way to get things going will help set expectations and begin to put your mind at ease. Getting the answers to these questions will bring you comfort in being clear on the needs of the child and their family. Feeling comfortable in your knowledge of the child's unique needs and how to fulfill them for their safety and well-being will build your T1D caregiving confidence.

- This is my first time caring for a child with type 1 diabetes. What should I know?

- I have cared for a child(ren) with type 1 diabetes before, but I know each child's diabetes is unique. What should I know about your child, specifically in relation to diabetes?

- Does your child have any allergies or dietary restrictions? If so, what are they?

- How independent is your child with their diabetes management tasks?

- Does your child wear an insulin pump and/or continuous glucose monitor (CGM)?

- In a school setting: does your child have a 504 plan, IHP (Individualized Health Plan), or IEP (Individualized

Education Plan)? If so, may we go over it? If not, we should get one started.

- In an overnight setting: does your child need overnight blood glucose checks? At what times?

- What supplies does the child need to keep with them at all times? Will he/she carry the supplies or is that my responsibility?

- Are there any special foods I can/should keep on hand?

- How comfortable is your child talking about type 1 diabetes with their peers? Do they prefer to be private about their diabetes?

Glossary

Basal insulin – "background insulin;" the long-acting insulin (Lantus or Levemir) in a MDI basal-bolus treatment regimen or consistent micro-dose amounts of short-acting insulin (Humalog, Novolog, or Apidra) used in pump therapy that maintains blood glucose levels around the clock, between meals, and during sleep

Basal rate – the amount of short-acting insulin necessary for an individual to receive consistent micro-dosing via pump therapy, measured in units per hour

Bolus – the dose of short-acting insulin administered by injection or pump for snacks or meals containing carbohydrates or correction doses; Humalog, Novolog, and Apidra are fast-acting insulins for the purpose of delivering a bolus

Carbohydrate counting – the system by which people with diabetes determine insulin dosing for snacks and meals; a unit of insulin is delivered per every X grams of carbohydrate being consumed

Celiac disease – genetic autoimmune disease where the consumption of the protein gluten damages the small intestine, resulting in nutrients not being absorbed into the body

Continuous Glucose Monitor (CGM) – device that measures blood glucose levels continuously in real-time by using a sensor inserted under the skin that sends data, through a transmitter, to a display for consistent monitoring and alarms to high and low threshold results

Correction factor – the amount of insulin needed to bring blood glucose levels back to target levels based on insulin sensitivity; measured by ratio in relation to one unit per number of blood glucose "points" to which that unit of insulin will lower the blood glucose number; also known as "insulin sensitivity factor"

Diabetic ketoacidosis (DKA) – life-threatening complication that occurs when a lack of insulin causes glucose to build up in the blood; when cells are unable to use glucose for energy, the body burns fat and muscle instead, producing ketones in the bloodstream, causing a dangerous metabolic imbalance

Endocrinologist – doctor that specializes in conditions of the endocrine system or hormonal issues, including but not limited to type 1 diabetes

Glucagon – the hormone released by the liver to help regulate blood glucose levels, mimicked by the powder-liquid solution contained in Glucagon emergency kits for use in situations of extreme hypoglycemic excursions (extremely low blood sugar)

Glucometer/Glucose meter – medical device that measures the amount of glucose present in the blood within a certain moment of time (with a certain error margin per US Food and Drug Administration [FDA] regulations)

Hyperglycemia – high blood glucose generally defined as 180-250 mg/dl or higher

Hypoglycemia – low blood glucose generally defined as 70 mg/dl or lower

Insulin pump – wearable medical device that enables the patient to receive insulin through infusion versus injection

Insulin to carb ratio - a single unit of insulin to carbohydrate amount is called insulin to carb ratio ("I:C"/carb ratio)

Lancing device – a reusable appliance used in combination with disposable lancets to collect samples for blood glucose monitoring

Macronutrient – nutrient that provides calories or energy (fat, protein, or carbohydrate)

Multiple Daily Injections (MDI) – a basal/bolus regimen where insulin is delivered by injection with either syringe or pen

Test strip – the consumable element of the blood glucose testing process; for use in compatible glucometers/glucose meters to absorb the blood sample for meter analysis

Type 1 diabetes – an autoimmune condition with no method of prevention, nor cure, that causes the body to attack the insulin production that normally takes place in the pancreas, creating the need to either inject or pump insulin into the body to resume processing carbohydrates into glucose for use by the brain and body for energy

T1D – shorthand for "type 1 diabetes;" may also refer to an individual living with type 1 diabetes

Type 2 diabetes – a metabolic condition in which the body has difficulty utilizing the body's naturally produced insulin properly, either due to insulin resistance or the circumstance that the body needs more insulin than the body is able to produce; treatment protocol often begins with diet and exercise, followed by oral medications, non-insulin injectables, long-acting insulin, and/or basal-bolus insulin regimen

Untethered pumping – a method of insulin pump use that involves the T1D receiving their basal insulin from a long-acting insulin injection instead of the steady micro-doses of fast-acting insulin throughout the day; the pump is used for bolus insulin only (food or corrections)

Made in the USA
San Bernardino, CA
06 June 2020

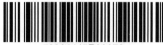